Procedure Checklists to Accompany
Craven and Hirnle's

Fundamentals of Nursing

HUMAN HEALTH AND FUNCTION

FIFTH EDITION

Procedure Checklists to Accompany
Craven and Hirnle's

Fundamentals of Nursing

HUMAN HEALTH AND FUNCTION

FIFTH EDITION

Elissa Swisher Sauer, RN, MSN

Adjunct Professor, Nursing
Assistant Dean Emerita, Division of Health Professions
Reading Area Community College
Reading, Pennsylvania

. Lippincott Williams & Wilkins
a Wolters Kluwer business

Philadelphia · Baltimore · New York · London
Buenos Aires · Hong Kong · Sydney · Tokyo

Managing Editor: Doris S. Wray
Senior Production Editor: Marian A. Bellus
Director of Nursing Production: Helen Ewan
Managing Editor / Production: Erika Kors
Art Director, Design: Joan Wendt
Art Director, Illustration: Brett MacNaughton
Senior Manufacturing Manager: William Alberti
Compositor: TechBooks
Printer: Victor Graphics

5th Edition

9 8 7 6 5 4 3 2 1

ISBN 0-7817-8604-5

Care has been taken to confirm the accuracy of the information presented and to
describe generally accepted practices. However, the author, editors, and publisher are
not responsible for errors or omissions or for any consequences from application of
the information in this book and make no warranty, express or implied, with respect
to the content of the publication.

The author, editors, and publisher have exerted every effort to ensure that drug
selection and dosage set forth in this text are in accordance with the current
recommendations and practice at the time of publication. However, in view of
ongoing research, changes in government regulations, and the constant flow of
information relating to drug therapy and drug reactions, the reader is urged to check
the package insert for each drug for any change in indications and dosage and for
added warnings and precautions. This is particularly important when the
recommended agent is a new or infrequently employed drug.

Some drugs and medical devices presented in this publication have Food and Drug
Administration (FDA) clearance for limited use in restricted research settings. It is the
responsibility of the health care provider to ascertain the FDA status of each drug or
device planned for use in his or her clinical practice.

LWW.com

Preface

This checklist manual will provide faculty and students with a portable handbook to the procedures in the text *Fundamentals of Nursing: Human Health and Function,* Fifth Edition. These checklists may be removed and used during supervision of students' performance of procedures. They may be modified to meet the needs of the situation, if desired. Students will find these checklists helpful when reviewing for the performance of various procedures.

The procedures in the checklists follow the steps of the procedures in the text. There are also subsets of procedures, for example, as in measuring weight. Otherwise, a separate checklist is provided for each procedure. In these instances, some of the introductory steps remain the same in each procedure but the subsequent steps vary. When this occurs, the procedure step number will deviate from the checklist step number even though the content is the same.

It is hoped that this manual will be useful to you, the faculty, as you teach and supervise students in the nursing classroom laboratory or in a clinical setting. It is also hoped that you, the students, will find the checklists useful in preparation for clinical experiences.

Elissa Swisher Sauer, RN, MSN

Contents

Procedure Checklists to Accompany Craven and Hirnle's Fundamentals of Nursing: Human Health and Function, 5th edition

Name _____ Date _____

Unit _____ Position _____

Instructor/Evaluator: _____ Position _____

Excellent	Satisfactory	Needs Practice	PROCEDURE 26-1 **Measuring Weight**	Comments
			Goal: Provide baseline data from which to assess total fluid balance or nutritional status and to determine drug dosages.	
____	____	____	1. Have client void before weighing.	
____	____	____	2. Have client wear same clothing for each weight measurement, and remove slippers or shoes.	
____	____	____	3. Place protective paper or cloth on scale.	
____	____	____	4. Check that scale registers zero. Adjust as necessary.	
			Weigh with Standing Scale	
____	____	____	1. Assist client onto center of scale platform. Instruct client not to lean or hold onto supports.	
____	____	____	2. Read digital display or adjust counterweights to determine client's weight.	
____	____	____	3. Assist client from scale, and record weight in client's record.	
			Weigh with Chair Scale	
____	____	____	1. Place scale beside client and lock wheels.	
____	____	____	2. Transfer client onto chair. If arm of chair is removable, unlock and remove before transfer. Lock back into place after transfer.	
____	____	____	3. Read digital display or adjust counterweights to determine client's weight.	
____	____	____	4. Transfer client back to bed or wheelchair.	
____	____	____	5. Clean scale according to agency policy. Return to proper location and plug in. Keep battery charged for next use.	
			Weigh with Bed Scale	
____	____	____	1. Elevate client's bed to level of stretcher scale.	
____	____	____	2. With one or two assistants, turn client on side with back toward the scale.	
____	____	____	3. Roll scale toward bed, lock wheels in place, and lower stretcher onto bed.	
____	____	____	4. Position folded stretcher under client. Roll client onto stretcher.	

Measuring Weight (*Continued*)

Excellent	Satisfactory	Needs Practice		Comments
			Goal: Provide baseline data from which to assess total fluid balance or nutritional status and to determine drug dosages.	
____	____	____	5. Attach stretcher arms to stretcher, and gradually elevate stretcher about 2 inches above mattress surface. Inform client before elevating. Reassure that he or she will not fall, but head may feel lower than body.	
____	____	____	6. Determine that stretcher is not touching any equipment. Lift drains and tubing away from stretcher.	
____	____	____	7. Read digital display for client's weight.	
____	____	____	8. Gradually lower stretcher to bed. Remove stretcher arms and transfer client off stretcher. Remove stretcher.	
____	____	____	9. Unlock bed scale wheels and move away from bed.	
____	____	____	10. Assist client to comfortable position.	
____	____	____	11. Clean stretcher and scale according to agency policy. Return to proper location and plug in to prepare for next use.	
____	____	____	12. Record weight and note any extra linen or equipment weighed with the client.	

*Procedure Checklists to Accompany Craven and Hirnle's Fundamentals
of Nursing: Human Health and Function,* 5th edition

Name _____   Date _____

Unit _____   Position _____

Instructor/Evaluator: _____   Position _____

Excellent	Satisfactory	Needs Practice	PROCEDURE 26-2 **Assessing the Neurologic System**	
			Goal: To obtain baseline information about the client's neurologic status, assess orientation to environment, and evaluate cognitive function.	**Comments**
____	____	____	1. Wash hands.	
____	____	____	2. Assemble equipment and provide privacy.	
			Cognitive-Sensory Assessment	
____	____	____	1. Assess the client's level of consciousness by asking direct questions that require a verbal response. Note appropriateness of response and emotional status.	
____	____	____	2. Evaluate client's speech patterns.	
____	____	____	3. Observe general appearance: hygiene, appropriateness of clothing to setting and weather.	
____	____	____	4. If responses are inappropriate, ask direct questions related to person, place, and time (e.g., "What is your name?" "Where are you right now?" "What city do you live in?" "What day is this?"). Be sure a communication or language problem is not causing client's inappropriate response.	
____	____	____	5. If client does not respond or inappropriately responds to orientation questions, give simple commands (e.g., "Squeeze my fingers" or "Wiggle your toes"). If there is no response to verbal commands, test response to painful stimuli by applying firm pressure on client's sternum or finger-nail bed with your thumb. Avoid pinching client's skin to elicit a pain response.	
____	____	____	6. Document cognitive and sensory assessment objectively by stating specific client responses to verbal or tactile stimulation. (Use of Glasgow Coma Scale helps charting of frequent level of consciousness testing.)	
____	____	____	7. Assess function of cranial nerves. a. I (Olfactory)—Ask client to identify different mild aromas, like vanilla, coffee, chocolate, cloves.	
____	____	____		
____	____	____	b. II (Optic)—Ask client to read Snellen chart. c. III (Oculomotor)—Assess pupil reaction to penlight (pupillary reflex).	

PROCEDURE 26-2
Assessing the Neurologic System (*Continued*)

Excellent	Satisfactory	Needs Practice	**Goal:** To obtain baseline information about the client's neurologic status, assess orientation to environment, and evaluate cognitive function.	Comments
⎯⎯	⎯⎯	⎯⎯	d. III—Assess direction of gaze by holding finger 18 inches from client's face. Ask client to follow finger up and down and side to side (extraocular eye movements).	
⎯⎯	⎯⎯	⎯⎯	e. IV (Trochlear)—Assess direction of gaze when testing cranial nerve II.	
⎯⎯	⎯⎯	⎯⎯	f. V (Trigeminal)—Lightly touch cotton swab to lateral sclera of eye to elicit blink.	
⎯⎯	⎯⎯	⎯⎯	g. V (cont.)—Measure sensation of touch and pain on face with cotton wisp and pin.	
⎯⎯	⎯⎯	⎯⎯	h. VI (Abducens)—Assess direction of gaze when testing cranial nerve III.	
⎯⎯	⎯⎯	⎯⎯	i. VII (Facial)—Ask client to smile, frown, raise eyebrows.	
⎯⎯	⎯⎯	⎯⎯	j. VII (cont.)—Ask client to identify different tastes on tip and sides of tongue: sugar, salt, lemon juice.	
⎯⎯	⎯⎯	⎯⎯	k. VIII (Auditory)—Assess ability to hear spoken word.	
⎯⎯	⎯⎯	⎯⎯	l. IX (Glossopharyngeal)—Ask client to identify different tastes on back of tongue (as in j).	
⎯⎯	⎯⎯	⎯⎯	m. IX (cont.)—Place a tongue blade on posterior tongue while client says "ah" to elicit gag response.	
⎯⎯	⎯⎯	⎯⎯	n. IX (cont.)—Ask client to move tongue up and down and side to side.	
⎯⎯	⎯⎯	⎯⎯	o. X (Vagus)—Assess with cranial nerve IX by observing palate and pharynx move as client says "ah."	
⎯⎯	⎯⎯	⎯⎯	p. XI (Spinal accessory)—Ask client to turn head side to side and shrug shoulders against resistance from examiner's hands.	
⎯⎯	⎯⎯	⎯⎯	q. XII (Hypoglossal)—Ask client to stick out tongue to midline, then move it side to side.	
⎯⎯	⎯⎯	⎯⎯	8. Assess sensory pathways.	
⎯⎯	⎯⎯	⎯⎯	a. Client's eyes should be closed during all sensory tests.	
⎯⎯	⎯⎯	⎯⎯	b. Apply stimuli to skin in a random unpredictable order while comparing one side of body with the other.	
⎯⎯	⎯⎯	⎯⎯	c. Client should verbally state when he or she feels a particular stimulus. If an area of altered sensation is detected, note which spinal cord segment is affected by referring to a dermatome chart.	

Excellent	Satisfactory	Needs Practice		Comments

PROCEDURE 26-2
Assessing the Neurologic System (*Continued*)

Goal: To obtain baseline information about the client's neurologic status, assess orientation to environment, and evaluate cognitive function.

9. Test pain sensation first by lightly touching pointed end and then blunt end of sterile toothpick to proximal and distal aspects of arms and legs.

10. Test temperature sensation by touching skin with vials of hot and then cold water. Client should identify hot versus cold sensation.

11. Lightly stroke proximal and distal aspects of client's arms and legs with a cotton applicator or ball. Ask client to state when and where each stroke is felt.

12. Apply a vibrating tuning fork to the distal interphalangeal joint of fingers and great toe. Ask client to state what is felt and when it stops. If client does not feel vibration, move tuning fork to next joint until sensation is felt.

Activity-Mobility Assessment

1. Inspect arm and leg muscles for atrophy, tremors, fasciculations, or other abnormal movements.

2. Assess strength of specific muscle groups by having client extend or flex individual joints against resistance provided by examiner's hands. Test biceps, triceps, wrist and leg muscles, and ankle. Evaluate for symmetry of same muscle groups.

3. Ask client to close eyes and hold arms in front of body with palms up. Hold position for 30 seconds and observe for pronation of hands or drifting of arms. Notice weaknesses on one or both sides.

4. Evaluate coordination and balance:
   a. Perform a series of rapid alternating movements (RAMs).
      (1) Have client pat upper thigh by rapidly alternating palm and back of hand.
      (2) With dominant hand, have client touch thumb to each finger on that hand as quickly as possible.
      (3) Have client use dominant forefinger to first touch your forefinger, then his or her nose. Instruct client to repeat this as many times as fast as he or she can.

PROCEDURE 26-2
Assessing the Neurologic System (*Continued*)

Goal: To obtain baseline information about the client's neurologic status, assess orientation to environment, and evaluate cognitive function.

Excellent	Satisfactory	Needs Practice		Comments
____	____	____	b. Romberg test—Ask client to stand with feet together, arms at sides. Have client maintain this position for 30 seconds with eyes open, then 30 seconds with eyes closed. Assess for swaying. Stay close to client in case he or she begins to fall.	
____	____	____	c. Ask client to walk across room. Observe gait for symmetry, rhythm, limping, shuffling, or other abnormalities.	
____	____	____	5. Assess deep tendon reflexes (biceps, triceps, patellar, Achilles) using the following technique:	
____	____	____	a. Compare symmetry of reflex on each side of body.	
____	____	____	b. Extremity to be tested should be completely relaxed and slightly extended.	
____	____	____	c. Reflex hammer is held loosely and allowed to swing freely into an arc.	
____	____	____	d. Tap tendon briskly.	
____	____	____	e. Document reflexes by grading responses 0 to 4+ on a stick figure, comparing bilaterally: 0: no response	
____	____	____	1+: diminished reflex	
____	____	____	2+: normal	
____	____	____	3+: brisker than normal	
____	____	____	4+: hyperactive	
____	____	____	f. In newborn and infant, assess rooting, sucking, Moro, and tonic neck reflexes.	
____	____	____	6. Document all findings according to agency policy.	

Procedure Checklists to Accompany Craven and Hirnle's Fundamentals of Nursing: Human Health and Function, 5th edition

Name _____   Date _____

Unit _____   Position _____

Instructor/Evaluator: _____   Position _____

Excellent	Satisfactory	Needs Practice	PROCEDURE 26-3 **Auscultating Heart Sounds**	Comments
			Goal: To assess normal and abnormal functioning of the heart valves and to detect cardiac problems.	
____	____	____	1. Wash hands, assemble equipment, and provide for privacy.	
____	____	____	2. Assist client to supine position, lifting gown to expose chest. May reexamine client in upright sitting position and in a left lateral position.	
____	____	____	3. Warm diaphragm of stethoscope by holding between hands for a few moments.	
____	____	____	4. Listen in mitral area using the diaphragm. Identify first and second heart sounds (S_1 and S_2). Count heart rate, noting whether rhythm is regular or irregular. If irregular, count heart rate for 1 full minute. Note if irregularity has a pattern or is unpredictable.	
____	____	____	5. Listen in aortic area using the diaphragm. Concentrate first on S_1, then S_2, noting whether splitting occurs. Shift concentration to systole and then diastole. Listen for extra sounds, such as murmurs.	
____	____	____	6. Listen in pulmonic area still using only the diaphragm. Concentrate on S_1, S_2, systole, and then diastole. Compare loudness of S_2 in the aortic and pulmonic areas.	
____	____	____	7. Move the diaphragm and listen to the tricuspid and mitral areas.	
____	____	____	8. Return to aortic area. Listen in aortic area, using bell of stethoscope. Concentrate on S_1, S_2, systole, and diastole.	
____	____	____	9. Repeat same process, using the bell in pulmonic, tricuspid, and mitral areas. Especially in mitral area, concentrate during diastole to detect presence of a third or fourth heart sound (S_3 and S_4). To increase ability to hear S_3 or mitral murmur, have client lie on left side while auscultating with bell. An S_3 often disappears when client sits up.	
____	____	____	10. Replace client's clothes. Assist to comfortable position.	
____	____	____	11. Record findings, describing intensity, quality, and location of sounds.	

Procedure Checklists to Accompany Craven and Hirnle's Fundamentals of Nursing: Human Health and Function, 5th edition

Name _____ Date _____

Unit _____ Position _____

Instructor/Evaluator: _____ Position _____

Excellent	Satisfactory	Needs Practice		Comments
			PROCEDURE 26-4 ## Auscultating Breath Sounds	
			Goal: To listen for breath sounds that may indicate the presence of airway obstruction or disease process.	
___	___	___	1. Wash hands, assemble equipment, and provide for privacy.	
___	___	___	2. Assist client to upright sitting position, removing gown to expose chest.	
___	___	___	3. Warm diaphragm of stethoscope by holding between hands for a short time.	
___	___	___	4. Ask client to breathe deeply and slowly through mouth.	
			Auscultate Anterior Chest	
___	___	___	5. Place diaphragm of stethoscope about 1 inch below the middle of the right clavicle, making sure it lies between the ribs. Listen to one full inspiration and exhalation. Repeat the process at the corresponding site on the left side.	
___	___	___	6. Note normal and adventitious breath sounds at each point on the chest as you proceed.	
___	___	___	7. Move stethoscope downward about 1.5 to 2 inches along midclavicular line. Note sounds; move stethoscope laterally to opposite side.	
___	___	___	8. Move stethoscope downward another inch or two along midclavicular line to fifth intercostal space; note sounds and then move to same spot on opposite side of chest.	
			Auscultate Posterior Chest	
___	___	___	9. Instruct client to lean forward and cross arms in front.	
___	___	___	10. Auscultate area 2 inches below shoulders and 2 inches to right of spine. Note sounds, and move to corresponding point on left.	
___	___	___	11. Move stethoscope directly downward 2 or 2.5 inches. Note sounds, then move stethoscope laterally and listen on right.	
___	___	___	12. Repeat process, moving downward 2 to 2.5 inches. Listen to corresponding opposite side.	

Excellent	Satisfactory	Needs Practice	PROCEDURE 26-4 **Auscultating Breath Sounds (*Continued*)**	
			Goal: To listen for breath sounds that may indicate the presence of airway obstruction or disease process.	**Comments**
____	____	____	13. Move stethoscope downward to area just below scapula. Listen on right and left. Listen laterally along lower rib cage.	
____	____	____	14. Replace client's clothes and assist to comfortable position.	
____	____	____	15. Discuss findings with client.	
____	____	____	16. Record assessment findings, being specific as to the description and location of adventitious sounds.	

Procedure Checklists to Accompany Craven and Hirnle's Fundamentals
of Nursing: Human Health and Function, 5th edition

Name _____ Date _____

Unit _____ Position _____

Instructor/Evaluator: _____ Position _____

Excellent	Satisfactory	Needs Practice	PROCEDURE 26-5 **Auscultating Bowel Sounds**	Comments
			Goal: To determine presence or absence of intestinal peristalsis.	
___	___	___	1. Wash hands, provide privacy and warm stethoscope diaphragm.	
___	___	___	2. Ask client when he or she last ate.	
___	___	___	3. Have client urinate before the examination.	
___	___	___	4. Assist client to a supine position with abdomen exposed.	
___	___	___	5. Visually divide the abdomen into four quadrants using the umbilicus as the central crossing landmark.	
___	___	___	6. Place stethoscope diaphragm in each of the four quadrants of the abdomen. Listen for pitch, frequency, and duration of bowel sounds at each site.	
___	___	___	7. If bowel sounds are not heard, listen for 3 to 5 minutes in all quadrants before concluding that they are absent.	
___	___	___	8. Proceed with rest of physical examination, or cover client's abdomen and assist to comfortable position.	
___	___	___	9. Document findings.	

Procedure Checklists to Accompany Craven and Hirnle's Fundamentals of Nursing: Human Health and Function, 5th edition

Name _____   Date _____

Unit _____   Position _____

Instructor/Evaluator: _____   Position _____

Excellent	Satisfactory	Needs Practice	PROCEDURE 27-1 **Assessing Body Temperature**	Comments
			Goal: To obtain baseline data for comparing future measurements, to assess for temperature alterations, or to evaluate temperature response to therapies.	
			Assessing Oral Temperature With an Electronic Thermometer	
___	___	___	1. Wash hands. Identify client and explain the procedure.	
___	___	___	2. Remove electronic thermometer from battery pack, and remove temperature probe from unit, noting digital display of temperature on screen (usually 34° C or 94° F).	
___	___	___	3. Securely attach disposable cover over temperature probe.	
___	___	___	4. Hold probe in sublingual pocket of client's mouth.	
___	___	___	5. Wait for a beep (usually 10–20 seconds), which indicates the estimated temperature. Watch to see if temperature continues to rise. When it stops, remove probe from client's mouth, noting the temperature displayed on the unit.	
___	___	___	6. Displace probe cover by pressing the probe release button as you hold the probe over a waste container.	
___	___	___	7. Return probe to storage place within the unit and the thermometer to the battery pack.	
___	___	___	8. Record temperature on vital sign documentation record. Discuss findings with client if appropriate.	
			Assessing Rectal Temperature With an Electronic Thermometer	
___	___	___	1. Wash hands. Don clean gloves. Identify client and explain procedure.	
___	___	___	2. Remove rectal (red) electronic thermometer from battery pack, and remove temperature probe from unit, noting digital display of temperature on screen.	
___	___	___	3. Securely attach the disposable cover over the temperature probe.	
___	___	___	4. Close bedroom door or bed curtains. Assist client to Sims' position with upper leg flexed. Expose only anal area.	

PROCEDURE 27-1
Assessing Body Temperature (*Continued*)

Goal: To obtain baseline data for comparing future measurements, to assess for temperature alterations, or to evaluate temperature response to therapies.

Excellent	Satisfactory	Needs Practice		Comments
——	——	——	5. Apply water-soluble lubricant liberally to thermometer probe tip.	
——	——	——	6. Separate client's buttocks with one gloved hand.	
——	——	——	7. Ask client to take a deep, slow breath. Insert thermometer into anus in direction of umbilicus 0.5 inch for an infant and 1.5 inches for an adult. Do not force.	
——	——	——	8. Hold in place until beep is heard. Obtain reading.	
——	——	——	9. Displace probe cover by pressing the probe release button as you hold the probe over a waste container. Remove gloves and wash hands.	
——	——	——	10. Return probe to storage place within the unit and the thermometer to the battery pack.	
——	——	——	11. Record temperature on vital signs documentation record. Discuss findings with client if appropriate.	

Assessing Axillary Temperature With an Electronic Thermometer

Excellent	Satisfactory	Needs Practice		Comments
——	——	——	1. Wash hands. Identify client and explain the procedure.	
——	——	——	2. Remove electronic thermometer from the battery pack, and remove the oral temperature probe from the unit, noting the digital display of temperature on the screen (usually 34° C or 94° F).	
——	——	——	3. Securely attach the disposable cover over the temperature probe.	
——	——	——	4. Close bedroom door or unit curtains; assist client to comfortable position, and expose axilla by removing clothing.	
——	——	——	5. Insert thermometer into middle of axilla; fold client's arm down, and place across chest.	
——	——	——	6. Wait for a beep that indicates the estimated temperature. Watch to see if temperature continues to rise. When it stops, remove the probe from the client's axilla, noting the temperature displayed on the unit.	
——	——	——	7. Follow steps 6 to 9 in Assessing Oral Temperature With Electronic Thermometer.	

Assessing Body Temperature (*Continued*)

Excellent	Satisfactory	Needs Practice		Comments

Goal: To obtain baseline data for comparing future measurements, to assess for temperature alterations, or to evaluate temperature response to therapies.

Assessing Temperature Using a Tympanic Membrane Thermometer

1. Wash hands. Identify client and explain procedure.

2. Remove tympanic thermometer from recharging base, and attach tympanic probe cover to sensor unit.

3. Insert probe into ear canal, making sure the probe fits snugly. Avoid forcing probe too deeply into ear. Pulling on pinna may help straighten ear canal, which permits better exposure of tympanic membrane. Rotate probe handle toward the jawline.

4. Activate the thermometer, and watch for the temperature readout, which is usually displayed within 2 seconds. Remove thermometer.

5. Eject sensor probe cover directly into waste container, and return tympanic thermometer to base for recharging. Store away from temperature extremes.

6. Record temperature on vital signs documentation record. Discuss findings with client if appropriate.

Procedure Checklists to Accompany Craven and Hirnle's Fundamentals of Nursing: Human Health and Function, 5th edition

Name _____   Date _____

Unit _____   Position _____

Instructor/Evaluator: _____   Position _____

Excellent	Satisfactory	Needs Practice	PROCEDURE 27-2 **Obtaining a Pulse**	
			Goal: To obtain baseline measurement of heart rate and rhythm or to evaluate heart's response to various therapies or medications.	**Comments**

Obtaining a Radial Pulse

___	___	___	1. Wash hands. Identify client and explain procedure.
___	___	___	2. Position client comfortably with forearm across chest or at side with wrist extended.
___	___	___	3. Place fingertips of your first three fingers along the groove at base of thumb on client's wrist.
___	___	___	4. Press against radial artery to obliterate pulse, then gradually release pressure until pulsations are felt.
___	___	___	5. Assess pulse for regularity and strength.
___	___	___	6. If pulse is not easily palpable, use Doppler:
___	___	___	a. Apply conducting gel to end of probe or to radial site.
___	___	___	b. Press "on" button and place probe against skin on pulse site. Reposition slightly using firm pressure until pulsating sound is heard.
___	___	___	7. If pulse is regular, count pulse for 30 seconds and multiply by two. If pulse is irregular, count for 1 full minute. Count initial pulse as zero.
___	___	___	8. Record pulse on vital signs record or computerized record.

Obtaining an Apical Pulse

___	___	___	1. Wash hands, identify client, and explain the procedure.
___	___	___	2. Position client in supine or sitting position with sternum and left chest exposed.
___	___	___	3. Warm diaphragm of stethoscope by holding in palm of hand for 5 to 10 seconds.
___	___	___	4. Insert the earpieces of stethoscope into ears, and place diaphragm over apex of client's heart.
___	___	___	5. Assess heartbeat for regularity and dysrhythmias.
___	___	___	6. If rhythm is regular, count the heartbeat for 30 seconds and multiply by two. Count for 1 full minute if rhythm is irregular. Count initial pulse as zero.

PROCEDURE 27-2
Obtaining a Pulse (*Continued*)

Excellent	Satisfactory	Needs Practice	**Goal:** To obtain baseline measurement of heart rate and rhythm or to evaluate heart's response to various therapies or medications.	**Comments**
――	――	――	7. Replace client's gown, and assist client to return to a comfortable position.	
――	――	――	8. Share results of assessment with client, if appropriate.	
――	――	――	9. Document pulse on vital signs record or computerized record. Specify in documentation that an apical pulse was obtained.	

Procedure Checklists to Accompany Craven and Hirnle's Fundamentals of Nursing: Human Health and Function, 5th edition

Name _____ Date _____

Unit _____ Position _____

Instructor/Evaluator: _____ Position _____

PROCEDURE 27-3
Assessing Respiration

Goal: To assess respiratory status by evaluating rate and quality or to evaluate influence of medications or therapies on respirations.

Excellent	Satisfactory	Needs Practice		Comments
____	____	____	1. Wash hands and identify client.	
____	____	____	2. After assessment of pulse, keep fingers resting on client's wrist, and observe or feel the rising and falling of chest with respiration. If client is asleep, gently place hand on client's chest to feel chest movement. **Do not** explain procedure to client.	
____	____	____	3. When one complete cycle of inspiration and expiration has been observed, look at second hand of watch and count the number of complete cycles. If rate is regular in an adult, count 30 seconds and multiply by two. In children under 2 years of age or adults with irregular rate, count for 1 full minute.	
____	____	____	4. If respirations are shallow and difficult to count, observe at the sternal notch.	
____	____	____	5. Note depth and rhythm of respiratory cycle.	
____	____	____	6. Discuss findings with client, if applicable.	
____	____	____	7. Document respiratory rate, depth, rhythm, and character.	

Procedure Checklists to Accompany Craven and Hirnle's Fundamentals of Nursing: Human Health and Function, 5th edition

Name _____ Date _____

Unit _____ Position _____

Instructor/Evaluator: _____ Position _____

PROCEDURE 27-4
Obtaining Blood Pressure

Goal: To evaluate the client's hemodynamic status by obtaining information about cardiac output, blood volume, peripheral vascular resistance, and arterial wall elasticity; and to obtain baseline measurement of blood pressure.

Excellent	Satisfactory	Needs Practice		Comments
___	___	___	1. Wash hands, and identify client. Explain procedure to client. Assist client to a comfortable position with forearm supported at heart level and palm up.	
___	___	___	2. Expose upper arm completely.	
___	___	___	3. Wrap deflated cuff snugly around upper arm with center of bladder over brachial artery. Lower border of cuff is 2 cm above antecubital space in an adult, nearer the antecubital space in an infant.	
___	___	___	4. If using mercury manometer, the manometer is vertical and at eye level.	
___	___	___	5. Palpate brachial or radial artery with fingertips. Close valve on pressure bulb, and inflate cuff until pulse disappears. Inflate 30 mm Hg higher. Slowly release valve, and note reading when pulse reappears.	
___	___	___	6. Fully deflate cuff, and wait 1 to 2 minutes.	
___	___	___	7. Place stethoscope ear pieces in ears. Palpate the brachial artery, and place stethoscope diaphragm or bell over site.	
___	___	___	8. Close bulb valve by turning clockwise. Inflate cuff to 30 mm Hg above reading where brachial pulse disappeared.	
___	___	___	9. Slowly release valve so pressure drops about 2 to 3 mm Hg per second.	
___	___	___	10. Identify manometer reading when first clear Korotkoff sound is heard.	
___	___	___	11. Continue to deflate, and note reading when sound muffles or dampens (fourth Korotkoff) and when it disappears (fifth Korotkoff). American Heart Association recommends noting the 4th Korotkoff sound for children, 5th for adults. Note all three readings in adults if 4th and 5th Korotkoff sounds are more than 10 mm Hg apart.	
___	___	___	12. Deflate cuff completely and remove from client's arm.	

PROCEDURE 27-4
Obtaining Blood Pressure (*Continued*)

Excellent	Satisfactory	Needs Practice	**Goal:** To evaluate the client's hemodynamic status by obtaining information about cardiac output, blood volume, peripheral vascular resistance, and arterial wall elasticity and to obtain baseline measurement of blood pressure.	Comments
____	____	____	13. Record blood pressure. Record systolic and diastolic in the form 130/80. If three readings are to be recorded, use the form 130/80/40. Abbreviate RA or LA to indicate right or left arm measurement.	
____	____	____	14. Assist client to comfortable position, and discuss findings with client, if appropriate.	
____	____	____	15. Document findings on client's record.	

Procedure Checklists to Accompany Craven and Hirnle's Fundamentals of Nursing: Human Health and Function, 5th edition

Name _____ Date _____

Unit _____ Position _____

Instructor/Evaluator: _____ Position _____

Excellent	Satisfactory	Needs Practice	PROCEDURE 27-5 **Assessing for Orthostatic Hypotension** **Goal:** To assess the compensatory status of the cardiovascular and autonomic nervous systems to changes in body position.	Comments
____	____	____	1. Wash hands. Identify client and explain procedure.	
____	____	____	2. Position client supine with head of bed flat for 10 minutes.	
____	____	____	3. Check and record supine blood pressure and pulse. Keep blood pressure cuff attached.	
____	____	____	4. Assist client to a sitting position with legs dangling over the edge of bed. Wait 2 to 4 minutes and check blood pressure and pulse rate. Waiting period is convenient time to auscultate client's lung fields.	
____	____	____	5. Assist client to standing position. Wait 2 to 4 minutes and check blood pressure and pulse rate. Be alert to signs and symptoms of dizziness.	
____	____	____	6. Assist client back to comfortable position.	
____	____	____	7. Record measurements and any symptoms that accompany the postural change. **Report** a drop of 25 mm Hg. In systolic pressure or a drop of 10 mm Hg. In diastolic pressure.	
____	____	____	8. Discuss findings with client, if appropriate.	

Procedure Checklists to Accompany Craven and Hirnle's Fundamentals
of Nursing: Human Health and Function, 5th edition

Name _____ Date _____

Unit _____ Position _____

Instructor/Evaluator: _____ Position _____

Excellent	Satisfactory	Needs Practice	PROCEDURE 28-1 **Handwashing**	Comments
			Goal: To prevent transfer of microorganisms from healthcare personnel to client and from client to healthcare personnel.	
____	____	____	1. Remove all rings except a plain wedding band. Push watch 4 to 5 inches above wrist.	
____	____	____	2. Turn on the water and adjust temperature to warm. Do not splash water or lean against the wet sink. Faucets may be controlled by your hands or may be operated by knee lever or foot pedals.	
____	____	____	3. Hold hands lower than elbows, and thoroughly wet hands and lower arms under running water.	
____	____	____	4. Apply soap and rub palms, wrists, and back of hands firmly with circular movements. Interlace fingers and thumbs, moving hands back and forth. Continue using plenty of lather and friction for 15 to 30 seconds on each hand. Timing of scrub may vary depending on purpose of wash and the amount of contamination.	
____	____	____	5. Clean under fingernails using fingernails of other hand and additional soap. Use orangewood stick if available.	
____	____	____	6. Rinse hands and wrists thoroughly with hands held lower than forearms.	
____	____	____	7. Dry hands and arms thoroughly with paper towel, wiping from fingertips toward forearm. Discard in proper receptacle.	
____	____	____	8. Turn off water using clean, dry paper towel on faucets.	

Procedure Checklists to Accompany Craven and Hirnle's Fundamentals of Nursing: Human Health and Function, 5th edition

Name _____ Date _____

Unit _____ Position _____

Instructor/Evaluator: _____ Position _____

Excellent	Satisfactory	Needs Practice	PROCEDURE 28-2 **Surgical Hand Scrub**	Comments
			Goal: To remove as many microorganisms from the hands as possible before a sterile procedure and to decrease the risk of infection for high-risk groups.	
____	____	____	1. Remove rings. Apply surgical attire (scrubs, shoe cover, cap or hood, face mask, and protective eye wear).	
____	____	____	2. Wash and rinse hands for initial wash.	
____	____	____	3. Open disposable brush impregnated with antimicrobial soap, and adjust water temperature to warm using water control lever.	
____	____	____	4. Wet hands and arms. Keep elbows bent so that hands remain higher than elbows. Water will flow down hands and off elbows.	
____	____	____	5. Use nail stick or cleaner to clean under nails of both hands.	
____	____	____	6. Wet scrub brush or apply antibacterial soap if not already impregnated in the brush.	
____	____	____	7. *Anatomic timed scrub:* Starting with the fingertips, scrub each anatomic area (nails, fingers each side and web space, palmar surface, dorsal surface, and forearm) for the designated amount of time according to agency policy (usually about 5 minutes). Scrub vigorously using vertical strokes. Repeat with other hand. **Or** *Counted brush stroke method:* Starting with the fingertips, scrub each anatomic area (nails, fingers each side and web space, palmar surface, dorsal surface, and forearm) for the designated number of strokes according to agency policy. Scrub vigorously using vertical strokes. Repeat with other hand.	
____	____	____	8. Do not touch faucet, clothing, or other objects. Avoid splashing. Rinse hands thoroughly under warm running water, keeping hands elevated to allow water to drain off at the flexed elbow.	
____	____	____	9. Keep hands held upward to allow water to drip from the elbow. Dry with sterile towel.	

Procedure Checklists to Accompany Craven and Hirnle's Fundamentals of Nursing: Human Health and Function, 5th edition

Name _____   Date _____

Unit _____   Position _____

Instructor/Evaluator: _____   Position _____

Excellent	Satisfactory	Needs Practice	PROCEDURE 28-3 **Applying and Removing Sterile Gloves**	Comments

Goal: To prevent transfer of microorganisms from hands to sterile objects or open wounds.

Applying Gloves

Excellent	Satisfactory	Needs Practice		
____	____	____	1. Wash hands.	
____	____	____	2. Remove outside wrapper by peeling apart sides.	
____	____	____	3. Place package on clean, flat surface above waist level. Open wrapper from the outside, keeping gloves on inside surface.	
____	____	____	4. Grasp inside edge of glove with thumb and first two fingers of dominant hand. Holding hands above waist, insert nondominant hand into glove. Adjust fingers inside glove after both gloves are on.	
____	____	____	5. Slip gloved hand underneath second gloved cuff still in package, and pull over dominant hand.	
____	____	____	6. Keeping hands above waist, adjust glove fit, touching only sterile areas.	

Removing Gloves

Excellent	Satisfactory	Needs Practice		
____	____	____	1. With dominant hand, grasp outer surface of nondominant glove just below thumb. Peel off without touching exposed wrist.	
____	____	____	2. Place ungloved hand under thumb side of second cuff and peel off toward fingers, holding first glove inside second glove. Discard into appropriate receptacle.	
____	____	____	3. Wash hands.	

Procedure Checklists to Accompany Craven and Hirnle's Fundamentals of Nursing: Human Health and Function, 5th edition

Name _____   Date _____

Unit _____   Position _____

Instructor/Evaluator: _____   Position _____

Excellent	Satisfactory	Needs Practice	PROCEDURE 28-4 **Donning a Sterile Gown and Closed Gloving**	Comments
			Goal: To apply attire necessary to carry out sterile procedures safely.	
____	____	____	1. Locate all surgical attire (scrubs, shoe covers, cap or hood, face mask, and protective eye wear), and perform the surgical hand scrub as described in Procedure 28-2.	
			Donning a Sterile Gown	
____	____	____	2. Grasp folded sterile gown at the neckline and step away from the sterile field. Allow gown to unfold gently, being careful that it does not touch the floor. The inside of the gown is toward the wearer.	
____	____	____	3. Holding the arms at shoulder level, grasp the sterile gown just below the neckband near the shoulders, and slide arms in the sleeves until the fingers are at the end of the cuffs but not through the cuffs.	
____	____	____	4. Have someone tie the back of the gown, taking care that only the ties are touched and not the sides or front of the gown.	
			Closed Gloving	
____	____	____	5. With fingers still within the cuff of the gown, open the inner sterile glove package and pick up the first glove by the cuff using your nondominant hand.	
____	____	____	6. Position the glove over the cuff of the gown so the fingers are in alignment, and stretch the entire glove over the stockinette cuff, being careful not to touch the edge of the stockinette cuff. Fingers remain within the cuff of the gown.	
____	____	____	7. Work the fingers into the glove, and pull the glove up over the wrist with the nondominant hand that still remains within the cuff of the gown.	
____	____	____	8. Use the sterile gloved hand to pick up the second glove, placing it over the stockinette cuff of the dominant hand and repeating the glove application process.	
____	____	____	9. Adjust gloves for comfort and fit, taking care to keep gloved hands above waist level at all times.	

Procedure Checklists to Accompany Craven and Hirnle's Fundamentals of Nursing: Human Health and Function, 5th edition

Name _____ Date _____

Unit _____ Position _____

Instructor/Evaluator: _____ Position _____

PROCEDURE 28-5

Preparing and Maintaining a Sterile Field

Excellent	Satisfactory	Needs Practice	**Goal:** To create an environment to prevent the transfer of microorganisms during sterile procedures and to ensure sterility of supplies and equipment.	Comments
____	____	____	1. Wash hands.	
____	____	____	2. Inspect all sterile packages for package integrity, contamination, or moisture.	
____	____	____	3. During entire procedure, never turn your back on the sterile field or lower your hands below the level of the field.	
			Opening a Sterile Drape	
____	____	____	4. Remove the sterile drape from the outer wrapper, and place the inner drape in the center of the work surface at or above waist level with the outer flap facing away from you.	
____	____	____	5. Touching the outside flap only, reach around (rather than over) the sterile field to open the flap away from you.	
____	____	____	6. Open the side flaps in the same manner using the right hand for the right flap and the left hand for the left flap.	
____	____	____	7. Lastly, open the innermost flap that faces you, being careful that it does not touch your clothing or any object.	
			Adding Sterile Supplies to the Field	
____	____	____	8. Prepackaged sterile supplies are opened by peeling back the partially sealed edge with both hands or lifting up the unsealed edge taking care not to touch the supplies with your hands.	
____	____	____	9. Hold supplies 10 to 12 inches above the field, allowing them to fall to the middle of the sterile field. Wrapped supplies are added by grasping the sterile object with one hand and unwrapping the flaps with the other hand.	
____	____	____	10. Grasp the corners of the wrapper with the free hand, and hold them against the wrist of the other hand while you carefully *drop* the object onto the sterile field.	

PROCEDURE 28-5

Preparing and Maintaining a Sterile Field (*Continued*)

Goal: To create an environment to prevent the transfer of microorganisms during sterile procedures and to ensure sterility of supplies and equipment.

Excellent	Satisfactory	Needs Practice		Comments

Adding Solutions to a Sterile Field

11. Read the solution label and expiration date. Note any signs of contamination.

12. Remove cap and place it with the inside facing up on a flat surface. Do not touch inside of cap or rim of bottle.

13. Hold bottle 6 inches above container on the sterile field, and pour slowly to avoid spills.

14. Recap the solution bottle, and label it with date and time of opening if the solution is to be reused.

15. Add any additional supplies and don sterile gloves (Procedure 28-2) prior to starting the procedure.

Procedure Checklists to Accompany Craven and Hirnle's Fundamentals of Nursing: Human Health and Function, 5th edition

Name _____ Date _____

Unit _____ Position _____

Instructor/Evaluator: _____ Position _____

Excellent	Satisfactory	Needs Practice	PROCEDURE 29-1 **Administering Oral Medications**	Comments
			Goal: To provide a safe, effective, economic route for administering medications.	
____	____	____	1. Wash hands.	
____	____	____	2. Arrange medication administration record (MAR) next to medication supply, medication trays, and cups.	
____	____	____	3. Prepare medications for only one client at a time.	
____	____	____	4. Remove ordered medications from supply. Compare label on medication with MAR or electronic medication administration record (EMAR), and check the five rights of medication administration. Scan bar code if using bar code medication administration (BCMA). If a discrepancy exits, recheck the client's chart and medication orders.	
____	____	____	5. Calculate correct drug dosage if necessary.	
____	____	____	6. Prepare selected medications.	
____	____	____	a. Unit dosage: Place packaged medications directly into medicine cup, or lay on tray without unwrapping.	
			b. Medications from a multidose bottle: Pour tablets or capsules into the container lid, and transfer into medicine cup. Return any extra tablets to the bottle.	
____	____	____	c. Medications from a bingo card: Snap the bubble containing the correct medication directly over the medicine cup. Do not touch medications.	
____	____	____	d. Swallowing difficulty: If client has trouble swallowing tablets, grind with mortar and pestle or other drug-crushing device until smooth. Mix powder in small amount of pudding or applesauce. Do not crush enteric-coated tablets or extended-release tablets.	
____	____	____	e. Liquid medications: Remove cap and place on countertop inside up. Hold bottle so label is against palm of hand. Fill until bottom of meniscus is at desired dosage. Discard excess poured liquid from cup into sink. Do not pour back into bottle.	
____	____	____	7. Take medication directly to client's room. Do not leave medication unattended.	

PROCEDURE 29-1
Administering Oral Medications (*Continued*)

Excellent	Satisfactory	Needs Practice	**Goal:** To provide a safe, effective, economic route for administering medications.	Comments
——	——	——	8. Compare name on MAR with name on client's identification bracelet, using two separate identifiers (e.g. name, medical record number, social security number, date of birth). Do not dispense medication if the client is not wearing an identification bracelet. Scan client's identification bracelet if using bar code medication administration.	
——	——	——	9. Complete any pre-administration assessment (i.e., blood pressure) required for the specific medication to be administered.	
——	——	——	10. Compare medication with MAR, and recheck the five rights of medication administration. If using unit-dose medications, unwrap the medication and place in the cup before checking the five rights of the next medication.	
——	——	——	11. Explain medication's purpose to client.	
——	——	——	12. Assist client to sitting position if necessary. Give medication cup and glass of water to client.	
——	——	——	13. If client is unable to hold the medication cup, place pill cup to lips and introduce medication into his or her mouth. If tablet or capsule falls on floor, discard and repeat preparation.	
——	——	——	14. Stay with client until he or she swallows all medications. Look inside client's mouth if the client is cognitively impaired or has difficulty swallowing to ensure client receives the ordered medications.	
——	——	——	15. Dispose of soiled supplies, and wash hands.	
——	——	——	16. Record time medication was administered and any pre-administration assessment data collected. For PRN medications, note the time post-administration assessments for effectiveness are due.	

Procedure Checklists to Accompany Craven and Hirnle's Fundamentals of Nursing: Human Health and Function, 5th edition

Name _____   Date _____

Unit _____   Position _____

Instructor/Evaluator: _____   Position _____

Excellent	Satisfactory	Needs Practice	PROCEDURE 29-2 **Administering Medication by Metered-Dose Inhaler (MDI)**	Comments
			Goal: To deliver premeasured dose of medication to the bronchial airways and lungs.	
____	____	____	1. Check medication order (see Procedure 29-1, Steps 1 to 5).	
____	____	____	2. Assemble medication canister, inhalation mouthpiece, and spacer device if needed. Attach the medication canister to the inhaler mouthpiece by inserting the metal stem into the long end of the mouthpiece. Shake the canister several times.	
____	____	____	3. Assist the client to sitting or standing position. Perform the second medication check of five rights.	
____	____	____	4. Ask client to breathe out through his or her mouth.	
____	____	____	5. Position the mouthpiece 1 to 2 inches from client's open mouth. Instruct the client to breathe in slowly through his or her mouth. As client starts inhaling, press the canister down to release one dose of the medication.	
____	____	____	6. Instruct client to hold his or her breath for 10 seconds, if possible.	
____	____	____	7. Wait at least 1 minute before administration of a second dose or inhalation of a different medication by MDI. Administer bronchodilators by MDI before other inhaled medications.	
____	____	____	8. Wash hands and clean mouthpiece. If steroid medication was administered, have client rinse mouth.	
____	____	____	9. Reassess ease of breathing, respiratory rate, accessory muscle use, and breath sounds.	
____	____	____	10. Document medication administration and client status before and after administration.	
			Modification for Using a Spacer With an MDI	
____	____	____	11. Attach spacer to inhalation mouthpiece. After exhaling, instruct client to place the mouthpiece in his or her mouth and close lips around the mouthpiece. Depress the medication canister and have client inhale. If client can't take and hold a deep breath, advise to take two or three short breaths to get all the medication from the spacer.	

Procedure Checklists to Accompany Craven and Hirnle's Fundamentals of Nursing: Human Health and Function, 5th edition

Name _____ Date _____

Unit _____ Position _____

Instructor/Evaluator: _____ Position _____

Excellent	Satisfactory	Needs Practice	PROCEDURE 29-3 **Withdrawing Medication From a Vial**	Comments
			Goal: To withdraw a precise amount of medication from a vial while maintaining asepsis.	
____	____	____	1. Check medication order, and compare the name of the ordered medication with the label on the medication vial (see Procedure 29-1, and complete Steps 1 to 5).	
____	____	____	2. Assemble needle and syringe, keeping needle sterile.	
____	____	____	3. Pick up vial. If medication has been reconstituted or is in suspension, place vial between the palms, rotating or rolling the vial back and forth. Do not shake.	
____	____	____	4. Remove metal cap from vial. Cleanse top of vial with alcohol wipe, and remove guard from needle.	
____	____	____	5. Pull back on barrel of syringe to draw in a volume of air equal to the volume of the ordered medication dose. Holding vial between thumb and fingers of the nondominant hand, insert needle through the rubber stopper into the air space—not the solution—in the vial, and inject air.	
____	____	____	6. Invert vial and withdraw the ordered dose of medication by pulling back on the plunger. Make sure needle is in the solution to be withdrawn.	
____	____	____	7. Expel air bubbles and adjust dose if necessary.	
____	____	____	8. Remove needle from vial, and cover the needle with guard.	
____	____	____	9. Wash hands.	

Procedure Checklists to Accompany Craven and Hirnle's Fundamentals of Nursing: Human Health and Function, 5th edition

Name _____ Date _____

Unit _____ Position _____

Instructor/Evaluator: _____ Position _____

Excellent	Satisfactory	Needs Practice	PROCEDURE 29-4 **Withdrawing Medication from an Ampule**	Comments
			Goal: To withdraw full dose of medication from an ampule safely while maintaining asepsis.	
____	____	____	1. Check medication order, and make sure the solution in the ampule matches the ordered solution (see Procedure 29-1, and complete Steps 1 to 5).	
____	____	____	2. Assemble needle and syringe. Filter needle may be used.	
____	____	____	3. Pick up ampule and flick its upper stem several times with a fingernail to release medication trapped in ampule's upper chamber.	
____	____	____	4. Wrap a sterile gauze pad or alcohol wipe around the neck of the ampule before breaking the neck with an outward snapping motion.	
____	____	____	5. Discard the broken neck appropriately, and prepare to withdraw medication from ampule using one of the following methods: a. Place ampule upright on a flat surface, insert needle in the solution, and withdraw the correct amount of medication by pulling up on the plunger without touching the needle to the glass rim.	
____	____	____	b. Invert the ampule or tilt it sideways. Insert the needle into the solution; pull back on the plunger, and withdraw the proper dose of medication.	
____	____	____	6. Remove needle from solution. Hold needle upright, inspect the syringe, and dispel any air that may have been drawn into the syringe. Make sure the syringe contains the correct amount of medication. Expel any extra medication into a container.	
____	____	____	7. Cover needle with guard, and change needle if filter needle was used. Discard ampule in sharps container.	
____	____	____	8. Wash hands.	

Procedure Checklists to Accompany Craven and Hirnle's Fundamentals
of Nursing: Human Health and Function, 5th edition

Name _____   Date _____

Unit _____   Position _____

Instructor/Evaluator: _____   Position _____

Excellent	Satisfactory	Needs Practice	PROCEDURE 29-5 **Drawing Up Two Medications in a Syringe**	
			Goal: To minimize the number of injections a client receives and to prevent contaminating one vial of medication with medication from the other vial.	**Comments**
____	____	____	1. Wash hands. Compare medications with MAR (see Procedure 29-1, and complete Steps 1 to 5).	
____	____	____	2. Cleanse tops of both vials with antiseptic swab.	
____	____	____	3. With syringe, aspirate volume of air equal to medication dose from first medication (Vial A).	
____	____	____	4. Inject air into Vial A, being careful that needle does not touch solution.	
____	____	____	5. Remove syringe from Vial A. Aspirate volume of air equal to the medication dose from second medication (Vial B). Inject air into Vial B.	
____	____	____	6. Invert Vial B, and withdraw required volume of medication into syringe. Expel all air bubbles, and withdraw needle from Vial B.	
____	____	____	7. Determine what total combined volume of medication would measure on syringe scale.	
____	____	____	8. Insert needle into Vial A, invert vial, and carefully withdraw required volume of medication (as in Step 6).	
____	____	____	9. Withdraw needle from Vial A, and replace needle guard.	
____	____	____	10. Check medication and dosage before returning or discarding vials.	
			Modification for Insulin	
____	____	____	1. Wash hands.	
____	____	____	2. When preparing insulin in suspension, gently rotate vials between palms of hands to mix the suspension.	
____	____	____	3. Follow Steps 2 to 8 above.	
____	____	____	4. Establish routine order for drawing up insulin. The short-acting insulin is drawn up first followed by the cloudy intermediate-acting insulin. Glargine (Lantus) cannot be mixed with other types of insulin.	

*Procedure Checklists to Accompany Craven and Hirnle's Fundamentals
of Nursing: Human Health and Function,* 5th edition

Name _____ Date _____

Unit _____ Position _____

Instructor/Evaluator: _____ Position _____

Excellent	Satisfactory	Needs Practice	PROCEDURE 29-6 **Administering Intradermal Injections**	Comments
			Goal: To administer medication into dermal tissue to screen for allergic (antigen-antibody) dermal reactions.	
____	____	____	1. Check medication order (see Procedure 29-1, Steps 1 to 5).	
____	____	____	2. Assemble needle and syringe.	
____	____	____	3. Remove needle guard, and withdraw medication from vial. (See Procedure 29-3).	
____	____	____	4. Identify client by two identifiers (name, medical record number, social security number, or date of birth). Scan ID bracelet if using bar code medication administration. Explain procedure to client. Repeat check of five rights.	
____	____	____	5. Select injection site that is relatively hairless and free from tenderness, swelling, scarring, or inflammation.	
____	____	____	6. Remove needle guard. Hold syringe in dominant hand. Gently pull skin distal to intended injection site taut with nondominant hand.	
____	____	____	7. Holding syringe from above, at a 10- to 15-degree angle (almost parallel to skin), gently insert needle, bevel up, until dermis barely covers bevel.	
____	____	____	8. Stabilize needle, then inject medication slowly over 3 to 5 seconds.	
____	____	____	9. Withdraw needle. Do **not** wipe or massage site.	
____	____	____	10. Do **not** recap needle. Dispose of syringe and needle in sharps container.	
____	____	____	11. Record time and site of injection according to agency protocol.	
____	____	____	12. Instruct client when to return for reading of response: 15 to 60 minutes after injection for allergy testing and usually 48 to 72 hours after injection for tuberculin skin testing.	

Procedure Checklists to Accompany Craven and Hirnle's Fundamentals of Nursing: Human Health and Function, 5th edition

Name _____ Date _____

Unit _____ Position _____

Instructor/Evaluator: _____ Position _____

Excellent	Satisfactory	Needs Practice	PROCEDURE 29-7 **Administering Subcutaneous Injections**	Comments
			Goal: To ensure more rapid absorption and action of a medication than can be achieved orally.	
____	____	____	1. Check medication order (see Procedure 29-1, Steps 1 to 5).	
____	____	____	2. Assemble needle and syringe.	
____	____	____	3. Remove needle guard, and withdraw medication from container (see Procedures 29-3 and 29-4).	
____	____	____	4. Identify client by two identifiers. Scan ID bracelet if using bar code medication administration. Explain procedure to client. Recheck five rights.	
____	____	____	5. Don gloves.	
____	____	____	6. Select injection site that is free from tenderness, swelling, scarring, and inflammation.	
____	____	____	7. Cleanse site with antiseptic swab in circular motion from center outward. Allow area to dry thoroughly.	
____	____	____	8. Remove needle guard. Hold syringe in dominant hand. Place nondominant hand on either side of injection site. Spread or bunch skin to stabilize site and identify subcutaneous tissue.	
____	____	____	9. Hold syringe between thumb and forefinger of dominant hand. Inject needle quickly at a 45- to 90-degree angle, depending on amount of subcutaneous tissue. Release bunched skin.	
____	____	____	10. Aspirate by slowly pulling back on plunger. If blood appears in syringe, withdraw needle, discard syringe, and prepare a new injection. Do not aspirate when administering heparin or insulin.	
____	____	____	11. If no blood appears, inject medication with slow, even pressure.	
____	____	____	12. Remove needle quickly while pressing antiseptic swab over site.	
____	____	____	13. Gently massage site with antiseptic swab.	
____	____	____	14. Assist client to position of comfort.	
____	____	____	15. Do **not** recap needle. Dispose of syringe and needle in sharps container.	
____	____	____	16. Wash hands.	
____	____	____	17. Record according to agency protocol.	

Excellent	Satisfactory	Needs Practice	

Goal: To ensure more rapid absorption and action of a medication than can be achieved orally.

Comments

Modification for Insulin Administration

1. Routine aspiration is not necessary.
2. Systematically rotate injection sites to prevent lipodystrophy and variable insulin absorption.
3. Instruct clients who self-administer insulin about not needing to cleanse site with alcohol before injection or to wear gloves.

Modification for Heparin Administration

1. The abdomen except for 1 to 2 inches on either side of umbilicus is most frequently used site.
2. Roll or gently bunch tissue between thumb and forefinger to ensure heparin is administered into subcutaneous tissue. Do not tightly pinch skin.
3. Because heparin is an anticoagulant, do not aspirate for blood return or massage skin after injection.
4. After injection, slowly and smoothly withdraw needle to prevent leakage into subcutaneous tissue.

Procedure Checklists to Accompany Craven and Hirnle's Fundamentals
of Nursing: Human Health and Function, 5th edition

Name _____ Date _____

Unit _____ Position _____

Instructor/Evaluator: _____ Position _____

Excellent	Satisfactory	Needs Practice	PROCEDURE 29-8 **Administering Intramuscular Injections**	Comments
			Goal: To administer medication deeply into muscle tissue, without injury to client.	
____	____	____	1. Check medication order (see Procedure 29-1, Steps 1 to 5). Assemble needle and syringe.	
____	____	____	2. Prepare needle, syringe, and medication by following appropriate steps in Procedure 29-3 or Procedure 29-4. If medication is known to be irritating to subcutaneous tissues, replace needle after withdrawing medication.	
____	____	____	3. Identify client by two identifiers. Scan ID bracelet if using bar code medication administration. Explain procedure to client.	
____	____	____	4. Don gloves. Assist client to a comfortable position, and expose only the area to be injected.	
____	____	____	5. Select appropriate injection site by inspecting muscle size and integrity. Consider volume of medication to be injected.	
____	____	____	6. Use anatomic landmarks to locate exact injection site.	
____	____	____	7. Cleanse site with antiseptic swab, wiping from center of site and rotating outward.	
____	____	____	8. Remove needle guard. Hold syringe between thumb and forefinger of dominant hand (like a dart). Spread skin at the site with nondominant hand.	
____	____	____	9. Insert needle quickly at a 90-degree angle to client's skin surface.	
____	____	____	10. Stabilize syringe barrel by grasping with nondominant hand. a. Aspirate slowly by pulling back on plunger with dominant hand.	
____	____	____	b. If no blood appears, inject medication slowly.	
____	____	____	c. If blood appears in syringe, remove needle, dispose of syringe, and prepare new dose of medication.	
____	____	____	11. Withdraw needle while pressing antiseptic swab above site.	
____	____	____	12. Gently massage site.	

Administering Intramuscular Injections (*Continued*)

			Goal: To administer medication deeply into muscle tissue, without injury to client.	**Comments**

Excellent	Satisfactory	Needs Practice		
___	___	___	13. Do **not** recap needle. Dispose of equipment in sharps container.	
___	___	___	14. Wash hands.	
___	___	___	15. Record medication and client response according to agency protocol.	

Variation for Air Lock Injection Technique

___	___	___	1. Withdraw desired volume of medication into syringe.
___	___	___	2. Draw in an additional 0.2 mL of air.
___	___	___	3. Check medication dose in syringe; expel excess amount of medication from syringe.
___	___	___	4. Redraw in 0.2 mL of air, and recheck dose accuracy.
___	___	___	5. Insert the needle entering the client at a 90-degree angle to the client's skin surface and the floor. Position the client so the proper anatomic landmarks can be located for the chosen site and still allow the needle to enter the client at a 90-degree angle to the floor; for example, when using either the ventrogluteal or deltoid sites, the client must be side-lying.

Variation for Z-Track Injection (for Medications for Deep IM Use)

___	___	___	1. When preparing injection site, pull skin and subcutaneous tissues about 1 to 1.5 inches to one side of the selected site.
___	___	___	2. Insert syringe at a 90-degree angle.
___	___	___	3. Aspirate and administer medication while continuing traction on skin.
___	___	___	4. Leave needle inserted an additional 10 seconds.
___	___	___	5. Simultaneously remove needle and release traction on skin.

Procedure Checklists to Accompany Craven and Hirnle's Fundamentals of Nursing: Human Health and Function, 5th edition

Name _____   Date _____

Unit _____   Position _____

Instructor/Evaluator: _____   Position _____

Excellent	Satisfactory	Needs Practice	PROCEDURE 29-9 **Administering Medication by Intravenous Bolus (Less than 5 Minutes)**	Comments
			Goal: To achieve high blood levels of a medication in a short time period.	
____	____	____	1. Check medication order (see Procedure 29-1, Steps 1 to 5).	
____	____	____	2. If medication has not been prepared and labeled by pharmacy, the nurse prepares the medication. Draw up ordered medication from vial or ampule. Read package insert for proper amount and solution for dilution. Label syringe with name of medication and dose. Remove needle and dispose of it properly.	
____	____	____	3. Identify client by two identifiers and recheck 5 rights. Scan client's ID bracelet if using bar code medication administration.	
____	____	____	4. Explain procedure to client.	
____	____	____	5. Don gloves.	
			Administering Medication Into an Existing Intravenous Line	
____	____	____	1. Select injection port in IV tubing closest to IV insertion site.	
____	____	____	2. Attach syringe to injection port.	
____	____	____	3. Occlude the IV tubing above the injection port by pinching the tubing.	
____	____	____	4. Inject medication slowly into the IV port at the prescribed rate. Use a watch to time administration rate.	
____	____	____	5. If IV medication and IV solution in tubing are incompatible, flush line with normal saline solution while occluding catheter above port. Administer medication at prescribed rate; reflush with 10 mL of sterile normal saline solution, and release occlusion.	

PROCEDURE 29-9

Administering Medication by Intravenous Bolus (Less than 5 Minutes) (*Continued*)

Goal: To achieve high blood levels of a medication in a short time period.

Excellent	Satisfactory	Needs Practice		Comments

Administering the Drug Into Intermittent Injection Device or Lock Device

1. Don gloves.
2. Attach syringe with 1 mL normal saline solution into injection port and flush. Remove syringe.
3. Attach syringe with medication into injection port. Inject medication slowly at the prescribed rate. Use watch to time safe administration rate. Remove syringe.
4. Attach syringe with 1 to 3 mL of normal saline into injection port and flush the port with saline.
5. Dispose of used syringes properly and wash hands.
6. Document medication administration.
7. Evaluate and chart client's response to medication therapy.

Procedure Checklists to Accompany Craven and Hirnle's Fundamentals of Nursing: Human Health and Function, 5th edition

Name _____   Date _____

Unit _____   Position _____

Instructor/Evaluator: _____   Position _____

Excellent	Satisfactory	Needs Practice	PROCEDURE 29-10 **Administering Intravenous Medications Using Intermittent Infusion Technique**	Comments
			Goal: To maintain therapeutic levels of medication in client's blood, dilute irritating intravenous solutions, or prevent combining incompatible medications.	
			Procedure When Using Syringe Pump and Heparin Lock	
___	___	___	1. Check medication order (see Procedure 29-1, Steps 1 to 5).	
___	___	___	2. Prepare the medication syringe and IV tubing. Examine the syringe for any air bubbles, and expel any that are present. Attach the syringe to the extension tubing, and gently push the syringe plunger to prime tubing. Cover adaptor.	
___	___	___	3. Secure the medication syringe into the pump with the flange of the syringe in the clamp's groove.	
___	___	___	4. Confirm client's identity by checking two identifiers. Scan client's ID bracelet if using bar code medication administration. Recheck the five rights, and explain the procedure to the client.	
___	___	___	5. Don gloves.	
___	___	___	6. Attach syringe with normal saline into the lock device. Flush lock with normal saline.	
___	___	___	7. Attach tubing to lock device. Secure IV tubing to IV site with tape.	
___	___	___	8. Program the pump for the appropriate infusion speed and press the start key. The medication syringe label often indicates the suggested infusion speed, typically 30 to 60 minutes. If uncertain, consult a drug reference handbook or pharmacist.	
___	___	___	9. Document medication administration.	
___	___	___	10. Assess client and infusion device 5 to 10 minutes after infusion has begun.	
___	___	___	11. When the completion alarm sounds, return to client's room and press the pump's stop key.	
___	___	___	12. Don gloves. Remove tubing from lock device. Attach syringe with 1 to 3 mL normal saline or heparin flush solution and flush lock.	

Excellent	Satisfactory	Needs Practice		Comments

Administering Intravenous Medications Using Intermittent Infusion Technique (*Continued*)

Goal: To maintain therapeutic levels of medication in client's blood, dilute irritating intravenous solutions, or prevent combining incompatible medications.

13. Replace lock with new sterile cap.
14. Dispose of syringes in proper container. Wash hands.

Administering Intermittent Intravenous Medication Into Primary Intravenous Line Using an EID

1. Check medication order. See Procedure 29-1, Steps 1 to 5.
2. Confirm client's identity using two identifiers and check five rights again.
3. Hang medication bag at or above level of primary IV solution. Insert secondary line into the adaptor port.
4. Check compatibility of medications to be administered with the IV solution being infused and any other infusing medications. If medications are not compatible with primary IV solution, clamp primary IV tubing above injection port, insert syringe with 20 mL of normal saline flush solution, and flush IV line. Do **not** administer IV medication through tubing that is infusing blood products or total parenteral nutrition.
5. Connect secondary line (piggyback) to injection port or "Y" site on IV tubing closest to IV insertion site.
6. Program EID with the correct volume and infusion rate for secondary infusion. Release clamps and press "Start".
7. When medication has infused, discard medication bag and tubing (or reserve for next medication infusion) according to agency guidelines.
8. Wash hands.
9. Document medication administration and add IV volume to IV intake.

*Procedure Checklists to Accompany Craven and Hirnle's Fundamentals
of Nursing: Human Health and Function,* 5th edition

Name _____   Date _____

Unit _____   Position _____

Instructor/Evaluator: _____   Position _____

Excellent	Satisfactory	Needs Practice	PROCEDURE 30-1 **Monitoring an Intravenous Infusion** **Goal:** To provide a safe, patent route for infusion of IV fluid therapy, ensure infusion of correct IV fluids and detect IV complications promptly.	Comments
____	____	____	1. Check physician's order for type of IV solution, additives, and infusion rate.	
____	____	____	2. Calculate hourly infusion rate or drops/min. or cc/hr when an EID is used.	
____	____	____	3. Compare IV fluid currently infusing with the ordered solution.	
____	____	____	4. Inspect the rate of flow at least every hour. For gravity-regulated IVs, check actual flow rate for 15 seconds and multiply by 4 for minute rate. Compare assessed rate with prescribed rate of flow. If infusion is ahead of schedule, slow it so the infusion will complete at the planned time. If infusion is behind schedule, review agency policy before increasing flow rate. Many agencies require a physician's order to increase the rate of flow. If electronic infusion device (EID) is used, the hourly infusion rate in milliliters per hour is programmed into the machine. Most EID manufacturers require use of cassette tubing unique to their machine.	
____	____	____	5. Inspect the system for leakage, and if present, locate the source. Tighten all connections within the system. If leak persists, slow IV flow rate to keep vein open, and replace tubing with sterile set.	
____	____	____	6. Inspect the tubing for kinks or blockages. Loosely coil tubing and place it on the bed.	
____	____	____	7. Inspect the infusion site for infiltration. This occurs when the needle becomes dislodged from the vein and IV fluid flows into the interstitial tissue. Look for signs of infiltration, including decreased rate of flow, swelling, pallor, coolness, and discomfort at or above the needle insertion site. If present, change the IV site. If a large amount of fluid infiltrated, elevate the arm above the heart on several pillows.	
____	____	____	8. Inspect arm above the insertion point for signs of phlebitis, including redness, swelling, warmth, and pain along the vein above the IV insertion site. If present, discontinue the IV and restart in another area.	

PROCEDURE 30-1
Monitoring an Intravenous Infusion (*Continued*)

Goal: To provide a safe, patent route for infusion of IV fluid therapy, ensure infusion of correct IV fluids and detect IV complications promptly.

Excellent	Satisfactory	Needs Practice		Comments
——	——	——	9. Inspect the insertion site for bleeding.	
——	——	——	10. Although monitoring IV therapy is a nursing responsibility, if client is able to comply, teach to contact the nurse if the following occur:	
——	——	——	a. The flow rate changes suddenly.	
——	——	——	b. The fluid container is almost empty.	
——	——	——	c. Blood is in the tubing.	
——	——	——	d. The site becomes uncomfortable.	
——	——	——	11. Chart any findings indicating complications of IV therapy (e.g., infiltration).	

Procedure Checklists to Accompany Craven and Hirnle's Fundamentals of Nursing: Human Health and Function, 5th edition

Name _____ Date _____

Unit _____ Position _____

Instructor/Evaluator: _____ Position _____

Excellent	Satisfactory	Needs Practice	PROCEDURE 30-2 **Changing Intravenous Solution and Tubing**	Comments
			Goal: To deliver IV therapy as ordered and decrease risk of client infection.	
			Changing Solution Container	
____	____	____	1. Review physician's orders for current IV fluid orders.	
____	____	____	2. Check label on currently infusing solution for date and time they were hung.	
____	____	____	3. Determine date and time of last tubing change. Review agency policy.	
____	____	____	4. Inspect IV system to determine type of tubing required.	
____	____	____	5. Gather supplies.	
____	____	____	6. Wash hands.	
____	____	____	7. Compare solution with physician's order. Adhere to five rights of medication administration.	
____	____	____	8. Remove IV bag from outer wrapper. Look for leaks or impurities in the bag.	
____	____	____	9. Label solution container with client's name, solution type, additives, date, and time hung. Check prelabeled container with physician's order. Line up time strip with volume amount on bag or bottle. Record solution change in the client's record.	
____	____	____	10. Prepare container for spiking: a. If solution is in a plastic bag, remove plastic cover from entry nipple. Maintain sterility of nipple end.	
____	____	____	b. If solution is in a bottle, remove metal cap, metal disk, and rubber disk. Maintain sterility of bottle top.	
____	____	____	11. Close clamp on the existing tubing.	
____	____	____	12. Take old solution container from pole and invert it.	
____	____	____	13. Remove spike from used container, maintaining its sterility. Spike new IV container with firm push/twist motion.	
____	____	____	14. Hang new container on IV pole.	

<table>
<tr><td>Excellent</td><td>Satisfactory</td><td>Needs Practice</td></tr>
</table>

PROCEDURE 30-2

Changing Intravenous Solution and Tubing (*Continued*)

Goal: To deliver IV therapy as ordered and decrease risk of client infection.

Comments

Excellent	Satisfactory	Needs Practice		
____	____	____	15. Inspect tubing for air bubbles, and assess that drip chamber is one-half full of solution.	
____	____	____	16. Adjust clamp to regulate flow rate or program EID, according to orders.	

Changing Solution and Tubing

Excellent	Satisfactory	Needs Practice		
____	____	____	1. Follow Steps 1 through 8 of Changing Solution Container.	
____	____	____	2. Open new tubing package, keeping protective covers on spike and catheter adapter.	
____	____	____	3. Adjust roller clamp on new tubing to fully closed position.	
____	____	____	4. Prepare new solution container as directed in Step 10 of Changing Solution Container.	
____	____	____	5. Remove protective cover from spike, maintaining sterility, and insert spike into new solution container.	
____	____	____	6. Hang container and "prime" drip chamber by squeezing gently, allowing to fill one-half full.	
____	____	____	7. Remove protective cap from catheter adapter, and adjust roller clamp to flush tubing with fluid. Replace protective cap.	
____	____	____	8. Adjust roller clamp on old tubing to close fully.	
____	____	____	9. Place towel or disposable underpad under extremity. Don clean, disposable gloves.	
____	____	____	10. Hold catheter hub with fingers of one hand (may use hemostat). With other hand, loosen tubing using gentle twisting motion. Remove old dressings if necessary.	
____	____	____	11. Grasp new tubing, remove protective catheter cap, and insert tightly into needle hub, while continuing to stabilize catheter hub with the other hand.	
____	____	____	12. Program EID or adjust roller clamp to start solution flowing according to physician's order.	
____	____	____	13. Remove and discard gloves.	
____	____	____	14. Secure tubing with tape.	
____	____	____	15. If dressing was removed, apply new dressing to IV site according to agency policy.	
____	____	____	16. Label new tubing with date, time, and your initials.	
____	____	____	17. Label solution container with client's name, solution type, additives, date, and time hung. Time label on side of IV container.	
____	____	____	18. Record solution and tubing change.	

Procedure Checklists to Accompany Craven and Hirnle's Fundamentals of Nursing: Human Health and Function, 5th edition

Name _____ Date _____

Unit _____ Position _____

Instructor/Evaluator: _____ Position _____

PROCEDURE 30-3
Converting to an Intermittent Infusion Device (IID) and Flushing

Goal: To maintain patency of intermittently used IV access.

Excellent	Satisfactory	Needs Practice		Comments
____	____	____	1. Check order for converting IV line to an intermittent infusion port.	
____	____	____	2. Identify all patient allergies.	
____	____	____	3. Assess site for signs of erythema, pain, tenderness, edema.	
____	____	____	4. Assess label and documentation for date and time of IV device placement.	
____	____	____	5. Gather supplies.	
____	____	____	6. Wash hands.	
____	____	____	7. Explain procedure to client.	
____	____	____	8. Prepare syringe with heparin flush solution or saline solution according to agency policy and manufacturer's recommendations for the type of device in place (may use between 0.5 and 1 mL [peripheral], 2.5 and 3 mL [central line] heparin flush, or 1 and 3 mL normal saline). Label syringes.	
____	____	____	9. Obtain appropriate IID.	
____	____	____	10. Don clean gloves.	

Converting IV to an Intermittent Infusion Device

Excellent	Satisfactory	Needs Practice		Comments
____	____	____	11. Clamp tubing of IV infusion with roller clamp.	
____	____	____	12. Hold the catheter hub firmly with your nondominant hand (a hemostat may be used if necessary). With dominant hand, quickly twist IV tubing to the left to loosen but not disconnect from IV catheter.	
____	____	____	13. Take IID out of package, keeping tip sterile. Hold in dominant hand between thumb and finger.	
____	____	____	14. Stabilize IV catheter with nondominant hand as you disconnect IV tubing. Quickly insert IID into IV catheter, twisting to the right to tighten.	
____	____	____	15. Tape IID to stabilize. Redress using transparent dressing if necessary.	

PROCEDURE 30-3

Converting to an Intermittent Infusion Device (IID) and Flushing (*Continued*)

Goal: To maintain patency of intermittently used IV access.

Excellent	Satisfactory	Needs Practice		Comments

Flushing With Needle Type System

1. Perform Steps 1 to 10 above.
2. Swab injection port with antiseptic swab and allow to dry.
3. Insert needleless syringe into the port, and aspirate gently for evidence of blood return.
4. Inject the recommended amount of saline or heparin flush using a pulsation technique, ending with 0.5 mL of solution remaining in syringe.
5. Dispose of uncapped needles and syringes in proper container.
6. Wash hands.
7. Document date, time, route, amount, and type of flush solution. Also document assessment of site.

Procedure Checklists to Accompany Craven and Hirnle's Fundamentals of Nursing: Human Health and Function, 5th edition

Name _____   Date _____

Unit _____   Position _____

Instructor/Evaluator: _____   Position _____

Excellent	Satisfactory	Needs Practice	PROCEDURE 30-4 **Administering Total Parenteral Nutrition (TPN)**	
			Goal: To provide parenteral nutritional support to selected clients.	**Comments**
			Monitoring Total Parenteral Nutrition Therapy	
____	____	____	1. Schedule and assist client with chest x-ray after central catheter insertion.	
____	____	____	2. Confirm correct solution is running at ordered rate. Check expiration date of solution. Use infusion controller to monitor and regulate flow rate. Infuse solutions with more than 10% dextrose or more directly into subclavian or internal jugular vein to dilute the solution rapidly and prevent thrombophlebitis.	
____	____	____	3. Inspect tubing and catheter connection for leaks or kinks. Tape all connections. Change tubing every 24 hours according to agency policy.	
____	____	____	4. Inspect insertion site for infiltration, thrombophlebitis, or drainage. If present, notify physician.	
____	____	____	5. Monitor vital signs, including temperature, every 4 hours.	
____	____	____	6. Assess for symptoms of air embolism: decreased level of consciousness, tachycardia, dyspnea, anxiety, "feeling of impending doom," chest pain, cyanosis, hypotension. If suspected, lay client on left side with head in Trendelenburg position.	
____	____	____	7. Use TPN line *only* for TPN and lipids. Never use for any other reason.	
____	____	____	8. Perform test for glucose every 6 hours. Notify physician if abnormal.	
____	____	____	9. Monitor laboratory tests of electrolytes, BUN, and glucose, as ordered, and report abnormal findings.	
____	____	____	10. Maintain accurate record of intake and output to monitor fluid balance.	
____	____	____	11. Weigh client daily and record.	
____	____	____	12. Inspect dressing once a shift for drainage and intactness. Change whenever loose or moist and at least every 48 hours.	

Administering Total Parenteral Nutrition (TPN) (*Continued*)

Excellent	**Satisfactory**	**Needs Practice**	**Goal:** To provide parenteral nutritional support to selected clients.	**Comments**

Administering Intralipids

1. Check solution against physician's order. Inspect solution for separation of emulsion into layers or for froth. Do **not** use if present.
2. Wash hands.
3. Attach fat emulsion tubing to bottle. Prime tubing as for conventional IV.
4. Identify client. Adhere to 5 rights of medication administration.
5. Identify Y-port on hyperalimentation tubing (below in-line filter).
6. Cleanse Y-port with antiseptic swab. Allow to dry. Insert connector into port. Secure with tape. *Note:* Lipids can be infused into a peripheral IV.
7. Adjust flow rate to infuse at 1 mL/min for adults and 0.1 mL/min for children. Infuse at this rate for 30 minutes while monitoring the client and vital signs every 10 minutes. Note: If any adverse reactions occur, stop infusion and notify physician.
8. If no adverse reactions occur, adjust flow rate:
   a. Adults: 500 mL intralipid over 4 to 6 hours.
   b. Children: up to 1 g/kg over 4 hours.
9. Document procedure according to agency policy.

Procedure Checklists to Accompany Craven and Hirnle's Fundamentals of Nursing: Human Health and Function, 5th edition

Name _____   Date _____

Unit _____   Position _____

Instructor/Evaluator: _____   Position _____

Excellent	Satisfactory	Needs Practice	PROCEDURE 30-5 **Administering a Blood Transfusion**	Comments
			Goal: To replace blood volume or blood components lost through trauma, surgery, or a disease process.	
____	____	____	1. Explain procedure to client. Have client sign consent form if required by agency policy.	
____	____	____	2. Obtain client's vital signs, including temperature.	
____	____	____	3. With another RN, an MD or other licensed staff at client's bedside, verify the blood component and the client's identity by comparing the laboratory blood record with the following:	
____	____	____	a. Client's name and identification number both verbally and against client's wrist band.	
____	____	____	b. Blood unit number on the blood bag label.	
____	____	____	c. Blood group and RH type on the blood bag label.	
____	____	____	d. Verify the type of blood component and the expiration date noted on the blood bag label.	
____	____	____	e. Document verification by both RN signatures on transfusion record.	
____	____	____	4. Wash hands.	
____	____	____	5. Open Y-type blood administration set, and clamp both rollers completely.	
____	____	____	6. Spike blood component unit bag port. Prime drip chamber and tubing with blood component.	
____	____	____	7. Spike 0.9% NaCl container with second spike. Keep roller clamp shut.	
____	____	____	8. Remove primary IV tubing from catheter hub, and cover end with sterile protector.	
____	____	____	9. Attach blood administration tubing to catheter hub and secure with tape.	
____	____	____	10. Open clamp to blood component. Open roller clamp below drip chamber and begin transfusion.	
____	____	____	11. Infuse blood slowly for first 15 minutes at 10 drops per minute.	
____	____	____	12. Observe and document condition during first 15 minutes, assessing for chilling, back pain, headache, nausea or vomiting, tachycardia, hypotension, tachypnea, or skin rash.	

Excellent	Satisfactory	Needs Practice	PROCEDURE 30-5 **Administering a Blood Transfusion (*Continued*)**	Comments
			Goal: To replace blood volume or blood components lost through trauma, surgery, or a disease process.	
____	____	____	13. If adverse reactions occur, close clamp to blood, open clamp to 0.9% NaCl, and notify physician immediately. Follow agency policy for laboratory notification and obtaining blood and urine specimens.	
____	____	____	14. If no adverse reactions occur after 15 minutes, regulate clamp to increase infusion according to physician's order. A unit of red blood cells is usually administered over 2 to 4 hours. Observe for signs or symptoms of transfusion reaction at least every 30 minutes throughout the transfusion. Obtain vital signs when observations warrant. Document observations in medical record.	
____	____	____	15. When blood transfusion is complete, clamp roller to blood and open roller to 0.9% NaCl solution. Infuse until tubing is clear (usually no more than 50 mL of normal saline).	
____	____	____	16. Obtain and document post-transfusion vital signs.	
____	____	____	17. If second blood component unit is to be transfused, slow 0.9% NaCl solution to keep vein open until next unit is available. Follow verification procedure and vital sign monitoring for each unit.	
____	____	____	18. If transfusion orders are complete, disconnect the blood administration tubing from catheter hub. Reconnect primary IV solution and tubing and adjust to desired rate.	
____	____	____	19. Wash hands.	
____	____	____	20. Document procedure on client's record.	

Procedure Checklists to Accompany Craven and Hirnle's Fundamentals of Nursing: Human Health and Function, 5th edition

Name _____ Date _____

Unit _____ Position _____

Instructor/Evaluator: _____ Position _____

Excellent	Satisfactory	Needs Practice	PROCEDURE 34-1 **Assisting with the Bath or Shower** **Goal:** To cleanse the skin, stimulate circulation, control body odors, and promote self-esteem.	Comments
____	____	____	1. Make sure tub and shower are clean.	
____	____	____	2. Prepare bathroom by placing towel or disposable bath mat on floor by tub or shower.	
____	____	____	3. Accompany or transport client to bathroom. Some clients may need to use shower chair for transportation.	
____	____	____	4. Place "occupied" sign on bathroom door.	
____	____	____	5. Keep client covered with bath blanket until water is ready.	
____	____	____	6. Fill bathtub halfway with warm water (105° F, 40.6° C). Test water or have client test water. If client is taking shower, turn shower on and adjust temperature.	
____	____	____	7. Help client into shower or tub, providing necessary assistance.	
____	____	____	8. Instruct client to use safety bars and call bell signal. Client may prefer to sit in shower chair to prevent fatigue.	
____	____	____	9. If client is unable to shower independently, stay with client at all times. Two nurses may be necessary with some clients.	
____	____	____	10. If client is showering or bathing independently, check on client within 15 minutes. Wash any areas he or she could not reach.	
____	____	____	11. Help client out of tub or shower. Assist with drying. If client is unsteady, drain water before getting client out of tub to prevent falls.	
____	____	____	12. Assist client with dressing and grooming.	
____	____	____	13. Help client to room. Return to bathroom to clean tub or shower according to agency policy. Discard soiled linen. Place "unoccupied" sign on door.	

Procedure Checklists to Accompany Craven and Hirnle's Fundamentals of Nursing: Human Health and Function, 5th edition

Name _____ Date _____

Unit _____ Position _____

Instructor/Evaluator: _____ Position _____

Excellent	Satisfactory	Needs Practice	PROCEDURE 34-2 **Bathing a Client in Bed**	Comments
			Goal: To cleanse the skin, stimulate circulation, control body odors, and promote self-esteem.	
____	____	____	1. Close curtains around bed or shut room door.	
____	____	____	2. Help client to use bedpan, urinal, or commode, if needed.	
____	____	____	3. Close window and doors to decrease drafts.	
____	____	____	4. Wash your hands.	
____	____	____	5. Raise bed to high position. Lock side rail up on opposite side of bed from your work.	
____	____	____	6. Remove top sheet and bedspread, and place bath blanket on client. Help client move closer to you, and remove gown. If client has an IV line, remove gown from arm, lower IV container, and slide it through gown with tubing. Rehang IV container and check flow rate. Note: If reusing top linen, place it on back of chair; otherwise, place in laundry bag.	
____	____	____	7. Lay towel across client's chest.	
____	____	____	8. Wet washcloth and fold around your finger to make a mitt.	
____	____	____	a. Fold washcloth in thirds.	
____	____	____	b. Straighten washcloth to take out wrinkles.	
____	____	____	c. Fold washcloth over to fit hand.	
____	____	____	d. Tuck loose ends under edge of washcloth on palm.	
____	____	____	<u>OR</u> Remove first cloth from bath bag packet.	
____	____	____	9. Cleanse eyes with water only, wiping from inner to outer canthus. Use separate corner of mitt for each eye.	
____	____	____	10. Determine if client would like soap used on face. Wash face, neck, and ears. Avoid letting soap sit in washbasin, or water will become too soapy for rinse. Liquid nondetergent cleansing agents, used in many agencies, do not require rinsing.	
____	____	____	<u>OR</u> Use first disposable cloth to cleanse face.	

Excellent	Satisfactory	Needs Practice	
			PROCEDURE 34-2 **Bathing a Client in Bed (Continued)**
			Goal: To cleanse the skin, stimulate circulation, control body odors, and promote self-esteem. **Comments**
———	———	———	11. Fold bath blanket off arm away from you. Place towel lengthwise under arm. Wash, rinse, and dry the arm using long firm strokes from fingers toward axilla. Wash axilla.
———	———	———	OR Continue to use disposable bag bath cloths as directed on package for cleansing parts of the body.
———	———	———	12. Repeat for arm and hand nearest you.
———	———	———	13. Apply deodorant or powder according to client's preferences. Avoid excessive use of powder or inhalation of powder.
———	———	———	14. Assess temperature of bath water, and change water if necessary. If you leave bedside, raise side rails to prevent accidental falls.
———	———	———	15. Place bath towel over chest. Fold bath blanket down to below umbilicus.
———	———	———	16. Lift bath towel off chest, and bathe chest and abdomen with cloth using long, firm strokes. Give special attention to skin under breasts and any other skin folds if client is overweight. Rinse and dry well. Apply light dusting of bath powder under breast or between skin folds.
———	———	———	17. Help client don a clean gown.
———	———	———	18. Expose leg away from you by folding over bath blanket. Be careful to keep perineum covered.
———	———	———	19. Lift leg and place bath towel lengthwise under leg. Wash, rinse, and dry leg using long, firm strokes from ankle to thigh to stimulate circulation and promote venous return.
———	———	———	20. Wash feet or place in basin of water as for hands. Rinse and dry well. Pay special attention to space between toes.
———	———	———	21. Repeat for other leg and foot.
———	———	———	22. Assess bath water for warmth. Change water if necessary.
———	———	———	23. Assist client to side-lying position. Apply gloves. Place bath towel along side of back and buttocks to protect linen. Wash, rinse, and dry back and buttocks. Give backrub with powder or lotion.

PROCEDURE 34-2
Bathing a Client in Bed (*Continued*)

Excellent	Satisfactory	Needs Practice	**Goal:** To cleanse the skin, stimulate circulation, control body odors, and promote self-esteem.	Comments
____	____	____	24. Assist to supine position. Assess if client can wash genitals and perineal area independently. If unable to, drape with bath blanket so that only genitals are exposed. Don disposable, clean gloves; using fresh water and a new cloth, wash, rinse, and dry genitalia and perineum.	
____	____	____	25. Complete care according to client's preference. Apply powder, lotion, and cologne.	
____	____	____	26. Assist with hair and mouth care.	
____	____	____	27. Make bed with clean linen.	
____	____	____	28. Clean equipment and return to appropriate storage area.	
____	____	____	29. Wash your hands.	
____	____	____	30. Chart significant observations.	

Procedure Checklists to Accompany Craven and Hirnle's Fundamentals of Nursing: Human Health and Function, 5th edition

Name _____ Date _____

Unit _____ Position _____

Instructor/Evaluator: _____ Position _____

Excellent	Satisfactory	Needs Practice	PROCEDURE 34-3 **Massaging the Back**	Comments
			Goal: To stimulate circulation to the skin and promote comfort and relaxation.	
⎯	⎯	⎯	1. Help client to side-lying or prone position.	
⎯	⎯	⎯	2. Expose back, shoulders, upper arms, and sacral area. Cover remainder of body with bath blanket.	
⎯	⎯	⎯	3. Wash hands in warm water. Warm lotion by holding container under running warm water.	
⎯	⎯	⎯	4. Pour small amount of lotion into palms.	
⎯	⎯	⎯	5. Begin massage in sacral area with circular motion. Move hands upward to shoulders, massaging over scapulae in smooth, firm strokes. Without removing hands from skin, continue in smooth strokes to upper arms and down sides of back to iliac crest. Continue for 3 to 5 minutes.	
⎯	⎯	⎯	6. While massaging, assess for broken skin areas and whitish or reddened areas that do not disappear. Do not apply pressure over areas of breakdown or redness.	
⎯	⎯	⎯	7. If additional stimulation is desired, can use pétrissage (kneading) over shoulders and gluteal area and tapotement (tapping) up and down spine can be done.	
⎯	⎯	⎯	8. End massage with long, continuous, stroking movements.	
⎯	⎯	⎯	9. Pat excess lubricant dry with towel. Re-tie gown and assist to comfortable position.	
⎯	⎯	⎯	10. Wash hands.	

Procedure Checklists to Accompany Craven and Hirnle's Fundamentals of Nursing: Human Health and Function, 5th edition

Name _____ Date _____

Unit _____ Position _____

Instructor/Evaluator: _____ Position _____

Excellent	Satisfactory	Needs Practice	PROCEDURE 34-4 **Performing Foot and Nail Care**	
			Goal: To maintain skin integrity around nails and maintain foot function.	**Comments**
____	____	____	1. Wash hands.	
____	____	____	2. Identify client. Help to chair if possible. Elevate head of bed for bedridden client.	
____	____	____	3. Fill washbasin with warm water (100°–104° F, 37.7°–40° C). Place waterproof pad under basin. Soak client's hands or feet in basin. Diabetic clients may soak feet for short period of time provided water is not too hot.	
____	____	____	4. Place call bell within reach. Allow hands or feet to soak for 10 to 20 minutes.	
____	____	____	5. Dry hand or foot that has been soaking. Rewarm water and allow other extremity to soak while you work on the softened nails.	
____	____	____	6. Gently clean under nails with orange stick. If nails are thickened and yellow, client may have fungal infection. Don disposable gloves and eye protection.	
____	____	____	7. Beginning with large toe or thumb, clip nail straight across. Shape nail with file. File rather than cut nails of clients with diabetes or circulatory problems.	
____	____	____	8. Push cuticle back gently with orange stick.	
____	____	____	9. Repeat procedure with other nails.	
____	____	____	10. Rinse foot or hand in warm water.	
____	____	____	11. Dry thoroughly with towel, especially between digits.	
____	____	____	12. Apply lotion to hands or feet. Do NOT apply lotion between toes of clients with diabetes.	
____	____	____	13. Help client to comfortable position.	
____	____	____	14. Remove and dispose of equipment.	
____	____	____	15. Wash hands.	

Procedure Checklists to Accompany Craven and Hirnle's Fundamentals of Nursing: Human Health and Function, 5th edition

Name _____   Date _____

Unit _____   Position _____

Instructor/Evaluator: _____   Position _____

PROCEDURE 34-5
Shampooing Hair of a Bedridden Client

Goal: To cleanse hair and scalp.

Excellent	Satisfactory	Needs Practice		Comments
——	——	——	1. Place waterproof pads under client's head and shoulders and remove pillow.	
——	——	——	2. Raise bed to highest position.	
——	——	——	3. Remove any pins from hair. Comb and brush hair thoroughly.	
——	——	——	4. Adjust bed to flat position. Place shampooing basin under head. Place bath towel around shoulders and folded washcloth where neck rests on basin.	
——	——	——	5. Fold bed linens down to waist. Cover upper body with bath blanket.	
——	——	——	6. Place waste basket with plastic bag under spout of shampoo basin on a chair or table at the bedside.	
——	——	——	7. Using water pitcher, wet hair thoroughly with warm water (approximately 110° F, 43.3° C). Check temperature by placing small amount of water on your wrist.	
——	——	——	8. Apply small amount of shampoo. Before shampooing, use hydrogen peroxide to dissolve matted blood in hair. Peroxide normally feels bubbly and warm. Reassure client it will not bleach the hair. <u>OR</u> Place hair on top of client's head. Place shampoo cap on top of hair and scalp. Work the lather into scalp and hair. No rinsing is necessary.	
——	——	——	9. Massage scalp with fingertips while making shampoo lather. Start at hairline and work toward neck.	
——	——	——	10. Rinse hair with warm water. Reapply shampoo and repeat massage.	
——	——	——	11. Rinse hair thoroughly with warm water. Clean hair "squeaks" when rubbed between fingers.	
——	——	——	12. Apply small amount of conditioner per client request. Rinse well.	
——	——	——	13. Squeeze excess moisture from hair. Wrap bath towel around hair. Rub to dry hair and scalp. Use second towel if necessary.	

Shampooing Hair of a Bedridden Client (*Continued*)

Excellent	Satisfactory	Needs Practice	**Goal:** To cleanse hair and scalp.	Comments
____	____	____	14. Remove equipment and wet towels from bed. Place dry towel around client's shoulders.	
____	____	____	15. Dry hair with hair dryer. Comb and style.	
____	____	____	16. Help client to comfortable position.	
____	____	____	17. Dispose of soiled equipment and linen.	

Procedure Checklists to Accompany Craven and Hirnle's Fundamentals of Nursing: Human Health and Function, 5th edition

Name _____   Date _____

Unit _____   Position _____

Instructor/Evaluator: _____   Position _____

Excellent	Satisfactory	Needs Practice	PROCEDURE 34-6 **Providing Oral Care**	Comments
			Goal: To cleanse tooth and mouth surfaces to prevent odor and caries.	
——	——	——	1. Wash hands.	
——	——	——	2. Close bedside curtains or room door, identify client, and explain procedure.	
——	——	——	3. Help client to a sitting position. If client cannot sit, help to a side-lying position.	
——	——	——	4. Place towel under client's chin.	
——	——	——	5. Moisten toothbrush with water. Apply small amount of toothpaste. If client is anticoagulated or has a clotting disorder, use very soft toothbrush or a sponge-ended swab to prevent gum bleeding.	
——	——	——	6. Hand toothbrush to client, or don disposable gloves and brush client's teeth as follows:	
——	——	——	a. Hold toothbrush at a 45-degree angle to gum line.	
——	——	——	b. Using short, vibrating motions, brush from gum line to crown of each tooth. Repeat until outside and inside of teeth and gums are cleaned.	
——	——	——	c. Cleanse biting surfaces by brushing with back and forth stroke.	
——	——	——	d. Brush tongue lightly. Avoid stimulating the gag reflex.	
——	——	——	7. Have client rinse mouth thoroughly with water and spit into emesis basin.	
——	——	——	8. Remove emesis basin, set aside, and dry client's mouth with washcloth.	
——	——	——	9. Floss client's teeth.	
——	——	——	a. Cut 10-inch piece of dental floss. Wind ends of floss around middle finger of each hand.	
——	——	——	b. Using index fingers to stretch the floss, move the floss up and down around and between lower teeth. Start at the back lower teeth and work around to other side.	
——	——	——	c. Using thumb and index fingers to stretch floss, repeat procedure on upper teeth.	
——	——	——	d. Have client rinse mouth thoroughly and spit into emesis basin.	
——	——	——	10. Dry client's mouth. Remove and dispose of supplies. Help client to comfortable position.	
——	——	——	11. Wash hands.	

Excellent	Satisfactory	Needs Practice	
			PROCEDURE 34-6

PROCEDURE 34-6
Providing Oral Care (*Continued*)

Goal: To cleanse tooth and mouth surfaces to prevent odor and caries.

Comments

Variations for the Unconscious Client

____ ____ ____ 1. Gather equipment.

____ ____ ____ 2. Place client in a side-lying position.

____ ____ ____ 3. Place towel or waterproof pad under client's chin.

____ ____ ____ 4. Place emesis basin against client's mouth, or have suction catheter positioned to remove secretions from mouth.

____ ____ ____ 5. Use padded tongue blade to open teeth gently. Leave in place between the back molars. Never put your fingers in an unconscious client's mouth.

____ ____ ____ 6. Brush teeth and gums as directed previously, using toothbrush or soft sponge-ended swab.

____ ____ ____ 7. Swab or suction to remove pooled secretions. A small bulb syringe or syringe without needle may be used to rinse oral cavity.

____ ____ ____ 8. Apply thin layer of petroleum jelly to lips to prevent drying or cracking.

Procedure Checklists to Accompany Craven and Hirnle's Fundamentals of Nursing: Human Health and Function, 5th edition

Name _____   Date _____

Unit _____   Position _____

Instructor/Evaluator: _____   Position _____

Excellent	Satisfactory	Needs Practice	PROCEDURE 34-7 **Using a Bedpan**	Comments
			Goal: To provide a means for elimination for clients who are confined to bed or unable to get to the bathroom or bedside commode.	
			Placing the Bedpan	
____	____	____	1. Wash hands. Don clean gloves.	
____	____	____	2. Close curtain around bed or shut door.	
____	____	____	3. Position and lock side rail up on opposite side of bed from which you work.	
____	____	____	4. Raise bed to height appropriate for nurse.	
____	____	____	5. For client who can raise buttocks and assist:	
____	____	____	a. Fold top linen down on nurse's side to expose client's hips.	
____	____	____	b. Have client flex knees and lift buttocks. Assist by placing your hand under sacrum, elbow on mattress, and lifting as a lever.	
____	____	____	c. Slide rounded smooth rim of regular bedpan under client. If using fracture pan, slide narrow flat end under buttocks.	
____	____	____	6. For client unable to assist by raising buttocks:	
____	____	____	a. Lower head of bed to flat position.	
____	____	____	b. Fold top linens down to expose client minimally.	
____	____	____	c. Help client roll to side-lying position.	
____	____	____	d. Place bedpan against buttocks and tucked down against mattress. Hold firmly in place and roll client onto back as bedpan positions under buttocks.	
____	____	____	7. Cover client with linen. Place call bell and toilet paper within reach.	
____	____	____	8. Raise head of bed 45 to 80 degrees unless contraindicated.	
____	____	____	9. Lower bed to lowest position. Place side rails up if indicated.	
____	____	____	10. Remove gloves. Wash hands. Allow client to be alone.	

Excellent	Satisfactory	Needs Practice	PROCEDURE 34-7 **Using a Bedpan (*Continued*)**	Comments
			Goal: To provide a means for elimination for clients who are confined to bed or unable to get to the bathroom or bedside commode.	

Removing the Bedpan

——— ——— ——— 11. Answer call bell promptly.

——— ——— ——— 12. Place soap, wet washcloth, and towel at bedside.

——— ——— ——— 13. Raise bed to appropriate working height for nurse.

——— ——— ——— 14. Fold back top linens to expose client minimally.

——— ——— ——— 15. Put on disposable clean gloves.

——— ——— ——— 16. Assess if client can wipe perineal area. If not, wipe area with several layers of toilet tissue. If specimen is to be measured or collected, dispose of soiled toilet tissue in separate receptacle, not bedpan. For female clients, wipe from urethra to anus.

——— ——— ——— 17. For client who can raise buttocks and assist with procedure:

——— ——— ———   a. Lower head of bed.

——— ——— ———   b. Have client flex knees and lift buttocks. Assist by placing one hand under sacrum and supporting bedpan with other hand to prevent spillage. Remove bedpan and place on bedside chair.

——— ——— ———   c. Offer soap, warm water, washcloth, and towel for client to wash hands or perineal area.

——— ——— ——— 18. For client unable to assist by raising buttocks:

——— ——— ———   a. Lower head of bed to flat position.

——— ——— ———   b. Fold top linen down to expose client minimally.

——— ——— ———   c. Help client to roll off bedpan and onto side. Use one hand to stabilize bedpan during turning to prevent spillage.

——— ——— ———   d. Wipe anal area with tissue. Wash perineum with soap and warm water. Pat dry.

——— ——— ——— 19. Assist client to comfortable position.

——— ——— ——— 20. Cover bedpan and remove from bedside. Obtain specimen if required. Empty and clean bedpan and return it to bedside.

——— ——— ——— 21. Remove and discard gloves. Wash hands.

——— ——— ——— 22. Spray air freshener if necessary to control odor, unless contraindicated (respiratory conditions, allergies).

Procedure Checklists to Accompany Craven and Hirnle's Fundamentals of Nursing: Human Health and Function, 5th edition

Name _____   Date _____

Unit _____   Position _____

Instructor/Evaluator: _____   Position _____

Excellent	Satisfactory	Needs Practice	PROCEDURE 34-8 **Making an Occupied Bed**	
			Goal: To provide clean linen for client who is unable to get out of bed.	**Comments**
____	____	____	1. Wash hands.	
____	____	____	2. Assemble equipment on bedside table or chair. Do **not** place on another client's bed.	
____	____	____	3. Close door or bedside curtains.	
____	____	____	4. Lock side rails up on side of bed opposite from where clean linen is stacked.	
____	____	____	5. Raise bed to comfortable working position. Lower side rail on your side of bed.	
____	____	____	6. Loosen all top linen from foot of bed. Remove bedspread and blanket separately. Without shaking, fold each and place over back of chair if they are to be reused. If they are soiled, hold them away from your uniform and place in linen bag.	
____	____	____	7. Leave top sheet on client or cover client with a bath blanket, then remove and discard top sheet.	
____	____	____	8. Loosen bottom sheet on your side. Lower head of bed to flat position. If client cannot tolerate flat position, lower head of bed as far as client can tolerate.	
____	____	____	9. Help client roll onto side facing away from you. Have client grasp side rail to assist. Additional personnel may be needed to assist with client positioning. Adjust pillow under head.	
____	____	____	10. Tightly fan-fold soiled draw sheet and tuck under buttocks, back, and shoulders. Repeat with soiled bottom sheet and tuck under client. Do not fan-fold mattress pad unless it is soiled.	
____	____	____	11. Place clean bottom sheet on bed. Unfold lengthwise so bottom edge is even with end of mattress and vertical center crease is at center of bed.	
____	____	____	12. Bring sheet's bottom edge over mattress sides and fanfold top of sheet toward center of mattress and place next to client. Tuck top edge of sheet under mattress. Miter the corner on your side: a. Grasp side edge of sheet about 18 inches down from mattress top.	

Excellent	Satisfactory	Needs Practice	PROCEDURE 34-8

PROCEDURE 34-8
Making an Occupied Bed (*Continued*)

Goal: To provide clean linen for client who is unable to get out of bed.

Comments

Excellent	Satisfactory	Needs Practice		Comments
___	___	___	b. Lay sheet on top of mattress to form a triangular, flat fold.	
___	___	___	c. Tuck sheet hanging loose below mattress under the mattress without pulling on the triangular fold.	
___	___	___	d. Pick up top of triangular fold, and place it over side of the mattress.	
___	___	___	e. Tuck this loose portion of sheet under the mattress.	
___	___	___	13. Tuck remaining portion of sheet under mattress. Note: If contour sheets are used, fit elastic edges under corner of mattress.	
___	___	___	14. Place draw sheet on bed with the center fold at center of bed. Position sheet so it will extend from client's back to below the buttocks. Fan-fold the top edge and place next to client. Tuck excess under mattress. Some agencies use a cloth waterproof pad instead of a draw sheet.	
___	___	___	15. Lock side rails up and move to other side of bed.	
___	___	___	16. Lower side rail. Help client roll over folds of linen onto other side. You may need additional help if client is unable to move easily.	
___	___	___	17. Move pillow under client's head.	
___	___	___	18. Remove soiled linen by folding into a square or bundle, with soiled side turned in. Place in linen bag.	
___	___	___	19. Grasp edge of fan-folded bottom sheet and pull from under client.	
___	___	___	20. Tuck top of sheet under top of mattress. Miter top corner.	
___	___	___	21. Facing bed, pull bottom sheet tight, and tuck excess linen under mattress from top to bottom.	
___	___	___	22. Unfold draw sheet by grasping at center. Tuck excess tightly under mattress. Tuck the middle first, then top, and finally the bottom.	
___	___	___	23. Help client to center of bed.	
___	___	___	24. Raise side rail if necessary, and move to side of bed where remainder of linen is stored.	
___	___	___	25. Place top sheet over client with center crease lengthwise at center of bed with seam side up. Unfold sheet from head to toe.	
___	___	___	26. Have client grasp top edge of clean top sheet. Remove bath blanket or soiled top linen by pulling from beneath clean top sheet.	

PROCEDURE 34-8
Making an Occupied Bed (*Continued*)

Excellent	Satisfactory	Needs Practice		Comments

Goal: To provide clean linen for client who is unable to get out of bed.

___ ___ ___			27. Discard in linen bag.
___ ___ ___			28. Smooth top sheet, with excess falling over bottom edge of mattress.
___ ___ ___			29. Spread blanket and bedspread evenly over bed. Miter the bottom corner, using all three layers of linen (sheet, blanket, bedspread). Leave sides untucked.
___ ___ ___			30. Move to opposite side of bed and miter bottom corner using all three layers of linen.
___ ___ ___			31. Standing at bottom of bed, grasp top covers about 10 inches from bottom of mattress. Loosen linen slightly by pulling on top covers or forming a pleat.
___ ___ ___			32. Put on clean pillowcases:
___ ___ ___			a. Grasp center of pillowcase with one hand on seamed end.
___ ___ ___			b. Gather case, turning it inside out over the hand holding it.
___ ___ ___			c. With same hand, grasp middle of one end of pillow.
___ ___ ___			d. Pull case over pillow with free hand.
___ ___ ___			e. Adjust case so corners fit over pillow.
___ ___ ___			33. Place pillows in center at head of bed.
___ ___ ___			34. Secure call bell within client's reach, and lower bed.
___ ___ ___			35. Arrange the bedside table, night stand, and personal items within easy reach.
___ ___ ___			36. Discard soiled linen and wash your hands.

Procedure Checklists to Accompany Craven and Hirnle's Fundamentals of Nursing: Human Health and Function, 5th edition

Name _____ Date _____

Unit _____ Position _____

Instructor/Evaluator: _____ Position _____

Excellent	Satisfactory	Needs Practice	PROCEDURE 35-1 **Using Body Mechanics to Move Clients**	Comments
			Goal: To prevent injury to the nurse's musculoskeletal system and to prevent injury to clients during transfer.	
____	____	____	1. Wash hands.	
____	____	____	2. Plan movement before doing it:	
____	____	____	a. Lock wheels on bed, stretcher, or wheelchair.	
____	____	____	b. Allow client to assist during move.	
____	____	____	c. Use mechanical aids (e.g., lifters, slide boards, body mobilizers) or additional personnel to move heavy clients.	
____	____	____	d. Slide, push, or pull client rather than lifting and carrying when possible.	
____	____	____	e. Tighten abdominal and gluteal muscles before lifting or moving client.	
____	____	____	f. Use smooth, rhythmic, coordinated movements.	
____	____	____	g. Plan movements before beginning when another person is assisting.	
____	____	____	3. Begin all movements with body aligned and balanced.	
____	____	____	a. Face client to be moved, and pivot your entire body without twisting your back.	
____	____	____	b. Place both feet flat on floor, bend knees slightly with one foot slightly in front of the other or one step apart.	
____	____	____	c. Bend knees to lower center of gravity toward client to be moved.	
____	____	____	4. When possible, elevate adjustable beds to waist level, and lower side rails.	
____	____	____	5. Carry objects close to body, and stand as close as possible to work area.	

Procedure Checklists to Accompany Craven and Hirnle's Fundamentals
of Nursing: Human Health and Function, 5th edition

Name _____ Date _____

Unit _____ Position _____

Instructor/Evaluator: _____ Position _____

Excellent	Satisfactory	Needs Practice	PROCEDURE 35-2 **Positioning a Client in Bed**	Comments
			Goal: To maintain proper body alignment for optimal ventilation and lung expansion, to maintain skin integrity, and to prevent musculoskeletal system deformities.	
			Moving a Client Up in Bed (One Nurse)	
____	____	____	1. Identify client and any positioning restrictions. Explain procedure and rationale to client.	
____	____	____	2. Lower head of bed to flat position, and raise level of bed to comfortable working height.	
____	____	____	3. Remove all pillows from under client. Leave one at head of bed.	
____	____	____	4. Instruct client to bend legs and put feet flat on bed.	
____	____	____	5. Place your feet in broad stance with one foot in front of the other. Flex your knees and thighs.	
____	____	____	6. Place one arm under client's shoulders and one arm under thighs. Keep head up and back straight.	
____	____	____	7. Rock back and forth on front and back legs to count of three. On third count, have client push with feet as you lift and pull client up in bed.	
____	____	____	8. Elevate head of bed and place pillows under head. Raise side rails and lower bed to lowest level.	
			Moving a Helpless Client Up in Bed (Two Nurses)	
____	____	____	1. Identify client and note any mobility restrictions. Explain procedure and rationale to client.	
____	____	____	2. Lower head of bed to flat position, and raise level of bed to comfortable working height.	
____	____	____	3. Remove all pillows from under client. Leave one at head of bed.	
____	____	____	4. One nurse stands on each side of bed with legs positioned for wide base of support and one foot slightly in front of the other.	
____	____	____	5. Each nurse rolls up and grasps edges of turn sheet close to client's shoulders and buttocks.	
____	____	____	6. Flex knees and hips. Tighten abdominal and gluteal muscles, and keep back straight.	

Excellent	Satisfactory	Needs Practice		Comments
			PROCEDURE 35-2 **Positioning a Client in Bed (*Continued*)**	
			Goal: To maintain proper body alignment for optimal ventilation and lung expansion, to maintain skin integrity, and to prevent musculoskeletal system deformities.	
——	——	——	7. Rock back and forth on front and back leg to count of three. On third count, both nurses shift weight to front leg as they simultaneously lift client toward head of bed.	
——	——	——	8. Elevate head of bed and place pillows under client's head. Adjust other positioning pillows as necessary. Put up side rails, and lower bed to lowest level.	
			Positioning Client in Side-Lying Position	
——	——	——	1. Identify client and note any mobility restrictions. Lower head of bed as flat as client can tolerate.	
——	——	——	2. Elevate and lock side rail on side client will face when turned.	
——	——	——	3. Using draw sheet, move client to edge of bed, opposite the side on which he or she will be turned.	
——	——	——	4. Place arm that client will turn toward away from his or her body. Fold other arm across chest.	
——	——	——	5. Flex client's knee that will not be next to mattress after turn. Have client reach toward side rail with opposite arm.	
——	——	——	6. Assume a broad stance with knees slightly flexed.	
——	——	——	7. Using a draw sheet, gently pull client over on side.	
——	——	——	8. Align client properly, and place pillows behind back and under head.	
——	——	——	9. Pull shoulder blade forward and out from under client. Support client's upper arm with pillow.	
——	——	——	10. Place pillow lengthwise between client's legs from thighs to foot.	
			Logrolling	
——	——	——	1. Obtain assistance of two or three other nurses.	
——	——	——	2. All nurses stand on same side of bed, with feet apart, one foot slightly ahead of the other. Flex knees and hips.	
——	——	——	3. Use one pillow to support client's head during and after turn.	
——	——	——	4. Place pillows between client's legs.	

PROCEDURE 35-2

Positioning a Client in Bed (*Continued*)

Excellent	Satisfactory	Needs Practice	**Goal:** To maintain proper body alignment for optimal ventilation and lung expansion, to maintain skin integrity, and to prevent musculoskeletal system deformities.	Comments
____	____	____	5. Instruct client to fold arms over chest and keep body stiff.	
____	____	____	6. Reach across client and support head, thorax, trunk, and legs. On count of three, roll client in one coordinated movement to lateral position.	
____	____	____	7. Support client in alignment with pillows as described in Side-Lying Position. Clients with suspected or known cervical spinal injuries should wear cervical collars to prevent injury to the spinal cord whenever turning or moving in bed.	

Procedure Checklists to Accompany Craven and Hirnle's Fundamentals of Nursing: Human Health and Function, 5th edition

Name _____   Date _____

Unit _____   Position _____

Instructor/Evaluator: _____   Position _____

Excellent	Satisfactory	Needs Practice	PROCEDURE 35-3 **Providing Range of Motion Exercises**	Comments
			Goal: To maintain joint mobility, improve or maintain muscle strength, and prevent muscle atrophy and contractures.	
——	——	——	1. Identify client and client's movement limitations. Explain procedure and purpose to client.	
——	——	——	2. Position client on back with head of bed as flat as possible. Elevate bed to comfortable working height.	
——	——	——	3. Stand on side of bed of joints to be exercised. Uncover only limb to be exercised.	
——	——	——	4. Perform exercises slowly and gently, providing support by holding areas proximal and distal to the joint. (Refer to Table 35-1 for illustrations of normal movement of each joint).	
——	——	——	5. Repeat each exercise five times. Discontinue or decrease ROM if client complains of discomfort or muscle spasm.	
——	——	——	6. Neck:	
——	——	——	a. Move chin to chest.	
——	——	——	b. Bend head toward back.	
——	——	——	c. Tilt head toward each shoulder.	
——	——	——	d. Rotate head in circular motion.	
——	——	——	e. Return head to erect position.	
——	——	——	7. Shoulder:	
——	——	——	a. Raise client's arm from side to above head.	
——	——	——	b. Abduct and rotate shoulder by raising arm above head with palm up.	
——	——	——	c. Adduct shoulder by moving arm across body as far as possible.	
——	——	——	d. Rotate shoulder internally and externally by flexing elbow and moving forearm so that palm touches mattress; then reverse the motion so that back of client's hand touches mattress.	
			e. Move shoulder in a full circle.	
——	——	——	8. Elbow:	
——	——	——	a. Bend elbow so that forearm moves toward shoulder.	
——	——	——	b. Hyperextend elbow as far as possible.	
——	——	——	9. Wrist and hand:	
——	——	——	a. Move hand toward inner aspect of forearm.	
——	——	——	b. Bend dorsal surface of hand backward.	

PROCEDURE 35-3
Providing Range of Motion Exercises (*Continued*)

Goal: To maintain joint mobility, improve or maintain muscle strength, and prevent muscle atrophy and contractures.

Excellent	Satisfactory	Needs Practice		Comments
_____	_____	_____	c. Abduct wrist by bending toward thumb.	
_____	_____	_____	d. Adduct wrist by bending toward fifth finger.	
_____	_____	_____	e. Make a fist, then extend the fingers.	
_____	_____	_____	f. Spread fingers apart, then together.	
_____	_____	_____	g. Move thumb across hand to base of fifth finger.	
_____	_____	_____	10. Hip and knee:	
_____	_____	_____	a. Lift leg and bend knee toward chest.	
_____	_____	_____	b. Abduct and adduct leg, moving leg laterally away from body and returning to medial position.	
_____	_____	_____	c. Internally and externally rotate hip by turning leg inward, then outward.	
_____	_____	_____	d. Take special care to support joints of larger limbs.	
_____	_____	_____	11. Ankle and foot:	
_____	_____	_____	a. Dorsiflex foot by moving foot so toes point upward.	
_____	_____	_____	b. Plantar flex by moving foot so toes point downward.	
_____	_____	_____	c. Curl toes down, then extend.	
_____	_____	_____	d. Spread toes apart, then bring together.	
_____	_____	_____	e. Invert by turning sole of foot medially.	
_____	_____	_____	f. Evert by turning sole of foot laterally.	
_____	_____	_____	12. Move to other side of bed and repeat exercises.	
_____	_____	_____	13. Reposition client to position of comfort.	
_____	_____	_____	14. Document ROM.	

Procedure Checklists to Accompany Craven and Hirnle's Fundamentals of Nursing: Human Health and Function, 5th edition

Name _____   Date _____

Unit _____   Position _____

Instructor/Evaluator: _____   Position _____

Excellent	Satisfactory	Needs Practice	PROCEDURE 35-4 **Assisting with Ambulation**	Comments
			Goal: To promote safe ambulation free of falls or injury.	
____	____	____	1. Identify client. Explain procedure and purpose of ambulation to client. Decide together how far and where to walk.	
____	____	____	2. Place bed in lowest position.	
____	____	____	3. Assist client to sitting position on side of bed. Assess for dizziness or faintness. Obtain orthostatic vital signs if complaints are present. Allow client to remain in this position until he or she feels secure.	
____	____	____	4. Help client with clothing and footwear.	
			One Nurse	
____	____	____	1. Wrap transfer belt around client's waist (optional according to assessment).	
____	____	____	2. Assist client to standing position, and assess client's balance. Return to bed or transfer to chair if very weak or unsteady. Be sure client does not grasp your neck for support, but places his or her hands around your shoulders or at your waist.	
____	____	____	3. Position yourself behind client while supporting him or her by waist or transfer belt.	
____	____	____	4. Take several steps forward with client, assessing strength and balance. Encourage client to use good posture and to look ahead, not down at feet.	
____	____	____	5. Ambulate for planned distance or time. If client becomes weak or dizzy, return to bed or assist to chair.	
____	____	____	6. If client begins to fall, place your feet wide apart with one foot in front. Support client by pulling his or her weight backward against your body. Lower gently to floor, protecting head.	
			Two Nurses	
____	____	____	1. Assist client to sitting position as described.	
____	____	____	2. Assist client to standing position with one nurse on each side.	

PROCEDURE 35-4
Assisting with Ambulation (*Continued*)

Excellent	Satisfactory	Needs Practice	

Goal: To promote safe ambulation free of falls or injury.   **Comments**

——— ——— ———   3. One nurse grasps the transfer belt to support the client. The other nurse may carry and manage equipment.

——— ——— ———   4. Walk with client using slow, even steps. Assess strength and balance. Encourage client to look forward rather than down at floor.

Using a Walker

——— ——— ———   1. Assist client to standing position. One hand remains on the arm of the chair or bed as client assumes an upright posture.

——— ——— ———   2. Have client grasp walker handles. Client moves walker ahead 6 to 8 inches placing all four feet of walker on floor. Client moves forward to walker.

——— ——— ———   3. Nurse should walk close behind and slightly to side of client.

——— ——— ———   4. Repeat above sequence until walk is complete.

Procedure Checklists to Accompany Craven and Hirnle's Fundamentals of Nursing: Human Health and Function, 5th edition

Name _____   Date _____

Unit _____   Position _____

Instructor/Evaluator: _____   Position _____

Excellent	Satisfactory	Needs Practice	PROCEDURE 35-5 **Helping Clients with Crutchwalking**	
			Goal: To increase client's level of activity safely after musculoskeletal injury.	**Comments**
			Four-Point Gait	
___	___	___	1. Instruct client to stand erect, facing forward in tripod position. Client places crutch tips 6 inches in front of feet and 6 inches to side of each foot.	
___	___	___	2. Client moves right crutch forward 6 inches.	
___	___	___	3. Client moves left foot forward to level of right crutch.	
___	___	___	4. Client moves left crutch forward 4 to 6 inches.	
___	___	___	5. Client moves right foot forward to level of left crutch.	
___	___	___	6. Repeat sequence.	
			Three-Point Gait	
___	___	___	1. Beginning in tripod position, client moves both crutches and affected leg forward.	
___	___	___	2. Client moves stronger leg forward.	
___	___	___	3. Repeat sequence. Client must bear entire weight on stronger leg to perform this gait.	
			Two-Point Gait	
___	___	___	1. Beginning in the tripod position, client moves left crutch and right foot forward.	
___	___	___	2. Client moves right crutch and left foot forward.	
___	___	___	3. Repeat sequence.	
			Swing-To Gait	
___	___	___	1. Client forms tripod position and moves both crutches forward.	
___	___	___	2. Client lifts legs and swings to crutches, supporting body weight on crutches.	

Excellent	Satisfactory	Needs Practice	
			PROCEDURE 35-5

PROCEDURE 35-5
Helping Clients with Crutchwalking (*Continued*)

Goal: To increase client's level of activity safely after musculoskeletal injury.

Comments

Swing Through Gait

1. Client forms tripod position and moves both crutches forward.
2. Client lifts legs and swings through and ahead of crutches, supporting weight on crutches.

Climbing Stairs

1. Use one crutch and the railing. Beginning in tripod position facing stairs, client transfers body weight to crutches and holds onto the railing.
2. Client places unaffected leg on stair.
3. Client transfers body weight to unaffected leg.
4. Client moves crutches and affected leg to stair.
5. Repeat sequence to top of stairs.

Procedure Checklists to Accompany Craven and Hirnle's Fundamentals of Nursing: Human Health and Function, 5th edition

Name _____   Date _____

Unit _____   Position _____

Instructor/Evaluator: _____   Position _____

Excellent	Satisfactory	Needs Practice	PROCEDURE 35-6 **Transferring a Client to a Stretcher**	Comments
			Goal: To transfer client without injury to client or nurse.	
——	——	——	1. Identify client. Explain procedure and purpose to client.	
——	——	——	2. Place stretcher parallel to bed. Raise bed to same level as stretcher. Lower side rails. Lock wheels on bed.	
——	——	——	3. One or two nurses stand on side of bed without stretcher. Two nurses stand on side of bed with stretcher.	
——	——	——	4. Loosen draw sheet on both sides of bed.	
——	——	——	5. Nurses on side without stretcher help client to move toward them onto his or her side, using draw sheet to pull client closer to stretcher.	
——	——	——	6. Nurses on stretcher side of bed slide transfer board under draw sheet and under client's buttocks and back.	
——	——	——	7. Slide client onto transfer board into supine position. Place client's arms across chest.	
——	——	——	8. Wrap end of draw sheet over curved end of transfer board, and slide client onto stretcher on count of three.	
——	——	——	9. Roll client slightly up onto side, and pull transfer board out from under him or her.	
——	——	——	10. Lock side rails up on bed side of stretcher, and move stretcher away from bed.	
——	——	——	11. Place sheet over client, and lock safety belts across client's chest and waist. Adjust head of stretcher according to client limitations.	

Procedure Checklists to Accompany Craven and Hirnle's Fundamentals
of Nursing: Human Health and Function, 5th edition

Name _____   Date _____

Unit _____   Position _____

Instructor/Evaluator: _____   Position _____

PROCEDURE 35-7
Transferring a Client to a Wheelchair

Goal: To increase mobility and independence by using wheelchair.

Excellent	Satisfactory	Needs Practice		Comments
____	____	____	1. Identify client and explain procedure.	
____	____	____	2. Position wheelchair at 45-degree angle or parallel to bed. Remove footrests and lock brakes.	
____	____	____	3. Lock bed brakes, lower bed to lowest level, and raise head of bed as far as client can tolerate.	
____	____	____	4. Assist client to side-lying position, facing the side of bed on which he or she will sit. Lower side rail, and stand near client's hips with foot near head of bed in front of and apart from other foot.	
____	____	____	5. Apply transfer belt. Grip belt to assist with transfer.	
____	____	____	6. Swing client's legs over side of bed. At the same time, pivot on your back leg to lift client's trunk and shoulders. Keep back straight, and avoid twisting.	
____	____	____	7. Stand in front of client, and assess for balance and dizziness.	
____	____	____	8. Help client to don robe and nonskid footwear.	
____	____	____	9. Spread your feet apart, and flex your hips and knees.	
____	____	____	10. Have client slide buttocks to edge of bed until feet touch floor.	
____	____	____	11. Rock back and forth until client stands on a count of three.	
____	____	____	12. Brace your front knee against client's weak knee as client stands.	
____	____	____	13. Pivot on back foot until client feels wheelchair against back of legs, keeping your knee against the client's knee.	
____	____	____	14. Instruct client to place hands on chair armrests for support. Flex your knees and hips as you assist client into chair.	
____	____	____	15. Adjust foot pedal and leg supports.	
____	____	____	16. Assess client's alignment in chair. Provide call light.	

Procedure Checklists to Accompany Craven and Hirnle's Fundamentals of Nursing: Human Health and Function, 5th edition

Name _____ Date _____

Unit _____ Position _____

Instructor/Evaluator: _____ Position _____

Excellent	Satisfactory	Needs Practice	PROCEDURE 35-8 **Transferring Client from Bed to Chair Using Hydraulic Lift** **Goal:** To safely transfer a client from bed to a chair when safe transfer is not possible without using a hydraulic lift.	Comments
____	____	____	1. Identify client and any mobility restrictions. Explain procedure and purpose to client.	
____	____	____	2. Place fabric sling evenly under client.	
____	____	____	3. Position hydraulic lift so the frame can be centered over the client. Attach the fabric sling to the frame. Note manufacturer's instructions for specifics of how sling should be attached to the frame.	
____	____	____	4. Have a nurse on each side of the hydraulic lift. Warn the client that he or she will be lifted from the bed. Support head and heavy casts as needed. Engage the hydraulic system to raise client from bed.	
____	____	____	5. Carefully wheel client in hydraulic lift away from the bed, supporting limbs as needed. Position over chair, and gently lower to chair using the hydraulic mechanism.	
____	____	____	6. The sling remains in place under the client and is reattached to the frame when the client is moved back to bed.	

Procedure Checklists to Accompany Craven and Hirnle's Fundamentals
of Nursing: Human Health and Function, 5th edition

Name _____   Date _____

Unit _____   Position _____

Instructor/Evaluator: _____   Position _____

Excellent	Satisfactory	Needs Practice	PROCEDURE 36-1 **Monitoring with Pulse Oximetry**	Comments
			Goal: To monitor arterial oxygen saturation (SaO$_2$) noninvasively and to detect deviations from normal promptly.	
____	____	____	1. Select appropriate type of sensor. A wide variety of sensors are available in sizes for neonates, infants, children, and adults. In addition, there are clip-on, adhesive, and disposable sensors. To select appropriate sensor, consider client's weight, level of activity, whether infection control is a concern, tape allergies, and the anticipated duration of monitoring.	
____	____	____	2. Explain purpose of procedure to client and family.	
____	____	____	3. Instruct client to breathe normally.	
____	____	____	4. Select appropriate site to place sensor. Avoid using lower extremities that may have compromised circulation or extremities receiving infusions or other invasive monitoring. Consider use of nasal sensor or forehead sensor for clients with poor tissue perfusion due to peripheral vascular disease or is receiving vasoconstrictor medications.	
____	____	____	5. Remove nail polish or acrylic nail from digit to be used.	
____	____	____	6. Attach sensor probe, and connect it to the pulse oximeter. Make sure the photosensors are accurately aligned.	
____	____	____	7. Watch for pulse-sensing bar on face of oximeter to fluctuate with each pulsation and reflect pulse strength. Double-check machine pulsations with client's radial or apical pulse.	
____	____	____	8. If continuous pulse oximetry is desired, set alarm limits on monitor to reflect high and low oxygen saturation and pulse rates. Ensure that the alarms are audible before leaving client. Inspect sensor site every 4 hours for tissue irritation or pressure.	
____	____	____	9. Read saturation on monitor, and document as appropriate with all relevant information on client's chart. Report SaO$_2$ less than 93% to physician.	

Procedure Checklists to Accompany Craven and Hirnle's Fundamentals of Nursing: Human Health and Function, 5th edition

Name _____   Date _____

Unit _____   Position _____

Instructor/Evaluator: _____   Position _____

Excellent	Satisfactory	Needs Practice	PROCEDURE 36-2 **Monitoring Peak Flow**	Comments
			Goal: To measure peak expiratory flow rate (PEFR) to assess respiratory function.	
____	____	____	1. Verify physician's order, and identify the client	
____	____	____	2. Explain the purpose of peak flow monitoring to client and family.	
____	____	____	3. Place indicator at base of numbered scale. Have client stand up.	
____	____	____	4. Tell client to take deep breath. Place meter in his or her mouth. Client should close lips around the mouthpiece. Remind client not to put tongue in the hole.	
____	____	____	5. Tell client to exhale as fast and as hard as he or she can, keeping a tight fit around the mouthpiece.	
____	____	____	6. Repeat Steps 3 through 5 twice more, and record the highest peak flow obtained in the three attempts.	
____	____	____	7. To determine "personal best" when beginning peak flow monitoring, obtain peak flow measurements in the morning and again in the evening over a 2-week period of good asthma control (feel good without any asthma symptoms). Client should take measurements before using bronchodilators.	
____	____	____	8. Healthcare provider will calculate zones based on percentage of personal best (green 80%–100%; yellow 50%–80%; red below 50%) and give instruction for what to do in each zone.	
____	____	____	9. Encourage client to comply with twice-a-day (morning and evening) peak flow monitoring before bronchodilator therapy and to follow healthcare provider's instructions for peak flows in each zone. Follow Steps 3 through 5.	

Procedure Checklists to Accompany Craven and Hirnle's Fundamentals of Nursing: Human Health and Function, 5th edition

Name _____   Date _____

Unit _____   Position _____

Instructor/Evaluator: _____   Position _____

Excellent	Satisfactory	Needs Practice	PROCEDURE 36-3 **Teaching Coughing and Deep Breathing Exercises** **Goal:** To facilitate respiratory functioning by increasing expansion, preventing alveolar collapse, and promoting expectoration of secretions.	Comments
			Deep Breathing	
____	____	____	1. Assist client to Fowler's or sitting position.	
____	____	____	2. Have client place hands palm down, with middle fingers touching, along lower border of rib cage.	
____	____	____	3. Ask client to inhale slowly through the nose, feeling middle fingers separate. Hold breath for 2 or 3 seconds.	
____	____	____	4. Have client exhale slowly through mouth. Repeat three to five times.	
			Controlled Coughing	
____	____	____	1. If adventitious breath sounds or sputum is present, have client take a deep breath, hold for 3 seconds, and cough deeply two or three times. Stand to client's side to ensure the cough is not directed at you. Client must cough deeply, not just clear the throat.	
____	____	____	2. If client has an abdominal or chest incision that will cause pain during coughing, instruct client to hold a pillow firmly over the incision (splinting) when coughing.	
____	____	____	3. Instruct, reinforce, and supervise deep-breathing and coughing exercises every 2 to 3 hours postoperatively.	
____	____	____	4. Document procedure.	

Procedure Checklists to Accompany Craven and Hirnle's Fundamentals of Nursing: Human Health and Function, 5th edition

Name _____   Date _____

Unit _____   Position _____

Instructor/Evaluator: _____   Position _____

Excellent	Satisfactory	Needs Practice	PROCEDURE 36-4 **Promoting Breathing with the Incentive Spirometer**	Comments
			Goal: To improve pulmonary ventilation and oxygenation and to loosen respiratory secretions.	
____	____	____	1. Verify the physician's order, and identify the client.	
____	____	____	2. Wash hands.	
____	____	____	3. Assist client to high Fowler's or sitting position.	
____	____	____	4. Determine the volume to set incentive spirometry goal based on calculated lung volumes. Use chart or have respiratory therapy calculate. Set volume indicator.	
			5. Instruct client in procedure:	
____	____	____	a. Seal lips tightly around mouthpiece.	
____	____	____	b. Inhale slowly and deeply through mouth. Hold breath for 2 or 3 seconds.	
____	____	____	c. Have client observe his or her progress by watching the balls elevate or lights go on, depending on type of equipment used.	
____	____	____	d. Exhale slowly around mouthpiece and breathe normally for several breaths.	
____	____	____	6. Repeat procedure 5 to 10 times every 1 to 2 hours per physician's orders.	

Procedure Checklists to Accompany Craven and Hirnle's Fundamentals of Nursing: Human Health and Function, 5th edition

Name _____ Date _____

Unit _____ Position _____

Instructor/Evaluator: _____ Position _____

Excellent	Satisfactory	Needs Practice	PROCEDURE 36-5 **Administering Oxygen by Nasal Cannula or Mask** **Goal:** To deliver low to moderate levels of oxygen to relieve hypoxia.	Comments
____	____	____	1. Review chart for physician's order for oxygen and ensure that it includes method of delivery, flow rate, duration of therapy.	
____	____	____	2. Wash hands. Identify client and proceed with 5 rights of medication administration.	
____	____	____	3. Explain procedure to client. Explain that oxygen will ease dyspnea or discomfort, and inform client concerning safety precautions associated with oxygen use. If client is using the cannula, encourage him or her to breathe through the nose.	
____	____	____	4. Assist client to semi or high Fowler's position if tolerated.	
____	____	____	5. Insert flowmeter into wall outlet. Attach oxygen tubing to nozzle on flowmeter; if using a high O_2 flow, attach humidifier.	
____	____	____	6. Turn on the oxygen at the prescribed rate. Check that oxygen is flowing through tubing.	

____	____	____	7. Cannula:
			  a. Place cannula prongs into nares.
			  b. Wrap tubing over and behind ears.
			  c. Adjust plastic slide under chin until cannula fits snugly.
			  d. If prongs dislodge from nares, replace promptly.	

____	____	____	8. Mask:
			  a. Place mask on face, applying from nose and over chin.
			  b. Adjust the metal rim over the nose, and contour the mask to the face.
			  c. Adjust elastic band around head so mask fits snugly.	

____	____	____	9. Assess for proper functioning of equipment, and observe client's initial response to therapy.	
____	____	____	10. Monitor continuous therapy by assessing for pressure areas on the skin and nares every 2 hours and rechecking flow rate every 4 to 8 hours.	
____	____	____	11. Document procedure and observations.	

Procedure Checklists to Accompany Craven and Hirnle's Fundamentals of Nursing: Human Health and Function, 5th edition

Name _____ Date _____

Unit _____ Position _____

Instructor/Evaluator: _____ Position _____

Excellent	Satisfactory	Needs Practice	PROCEDURE 36-6 **Monitoring a Client with a Chest Drainage System**	
			Goal: To monitor respiratory status of client with a chest tube and to ensure that the drainage system is functioning adequately.	**Comments**
____	____	____	1. Confirm physician's order, including amount of suction.	
____	____	____	2. Assist client to semi or high Fowler's position.	
____	____	____	3. Assess insertion site of chest tube. Note and document amount and color of drainage on dressing around insertion site. Feel insertion site for crepitus. Document any crepitus found. Reinforce insertion dressing as needed.	
____	____	____	4. Assess status of chest tubing. Be sure tubing remains at level of client and no dependent loops are present. Assess that there are no visible clots in tubing. You may gently "milk" (compress tubing with fingers) the clots to encourage movement into the drainage system, but never strip chest tubing.	
____	____	____	5. Assess drainage collection chamber. Be sure to keep chest drainage system upright. Assess for amount, color, and character of drainage. Mark collection chamber to reflect accurately amount of drainage accumulated during your shift. Note any sudden significant increase in amount of drainage.	
____	____	____	6. Assess suction chamber. Make sure the water level in suction chamber is at the prescribed amount of suction and that it is connected to the wall suction, which is turned on to continuous suction. Usually suction is set at 10–20 mm Hg.	
____	____	____	7. Assess system for air leaks. Check all external connections (i.e., chest tube connection to drainage system, suction tubing connection to drainage system). Examine water seal chamber as client breathes normally and as client coughs.	
____	____	____	8. Encourage client to cough, deep breathe, and use an incentive spirometer frequently. Provide analgesics as necessary. Note: Clamping of chest tubes is no longer recommended.	

Excellent	Satisfactory	Needs Practice	PROCEDURE 36-6 **Monitoring a Client with a Chest Drainage System (*Continued*)**	
			Goal: To monitor respiratory status of client with a chest tube and to ensure that the drainage system is functioning adequately.	**Comments**
____	____	____	9. If chest tube becomes expelled, do not leave client. Cover opening where chest tube was inserted with sterile 4×4 gauze, and keep direct pressure on the site. Send a colleague to call the physician immediately.	
____	____	____	10. Document chest tube drainage, patency of chest tubes, the presence of an air leak, the amount of suction, pain level, status of the dressing, and respiratory status.	

Procedure Checklists to Accompany Craven and Hirnle's Fundamentals of Nursing: Human Health and Function, 5th edition

Name _____ Date _____

Unit _____ Position _____

Instructor/Evaluator: _____ Position _____

Excellent	Satisfactory	Needs Practice	PROCEDURE 36-7 **Providing Tracheostomy Care**	Comments
			Goal: To maintain airway patency by removing mucus and encrusted secretions and to prevent infection or skin breakdown at stoma site.	
____	____	____	1. Verify physician's order, and identify client.	
____	____	____	2. Wash hands and don gloves.	
____	____	____	3. Explain procedure to client. Place client in semi to high Fowler's position.	
____	____	____	4. Suction tracheostomy tube. Before discarding gloves, remove soiled tracheostomy dressing, and discard with catheter inside glove. Note: Follow Procedure 36-8, suction secretions from airways. When suctioning through a tracheostomy tube insert catheter about 10 to 12 cm in an adult.	
____	____	____	5. Replace oxygen or humidification source, and encourage client to deep breathe as you prepare sterile supplies.	
____	____	____	6. Open sterile tracheostomy kit. Don sterile gloves. Pour normal saline into one basin and hydrogen peroxide into the second. Open several sterile cotton-tipped applicators and one sterile precut tracheostomy dressing, and place on sterile field. If kit does not contain tracheostomy ties, cut two 15-inch pieces of twill tape and set aside.	
____	____	____	7. Remove oxygen or humidity source. Note: For tracheostomy tube with inner cannula, complete Steps 7 to 25. For tracheostomy tube without inner cannula or plugged with a button, complete Steps 13 to 25.	
____	____	____	8. Unplug inner cannula by turning counterclockwise. Remove inner cannula.	
____	____	____	9. Place inner cannula in basin with hydrogen peroxide.	
____	____	____	10. Replace oxygen source over or near outer cannula. (Not all clients may require oxygen during tracheostomy care).	
____	____	____	11. Clean lumen and sides of inner cannula using pipe cleaners or sterile brush.	
____	____	____	12. Rinse inner cannula thoroughly by agitating in normal saline for several seconds.	

PROCEDURE 36-7
Providing Tracheostomy Care (*Continued*)

Excellent	Satisfactory	Needs Practice		Comments
			Goal: To maintain airway patency by removing mucus and encrusted secretions and to prevent infection or skin breakdown at stoma site.	
___	___	___	13. Remove oxygen source and replace inner cannula into outer cannula. "Lock" by turning clockwise until the two blue dots align. Replace oxygen or humidity source.	
___	___	___	14. Clean stoma under faceplate with circular motion using hydrogen peroxide-soaked cotton applicators. Clean dried secretions from all exposed outer cannula surfaces.	
___	___	___	15. Remove foaming secretions using normal saline-soaked cotton-tipped applicators.	
___	___	___	16. Pat moist surfaces dry with 4×4-inch gauze.	
___	___	___	17. Place dry, sterile, precut tracheostomy dressing around tracheostomy stoma and under faceplate. Do not use cut 4×4-inch gauze.	
___	___	___	18. If tracheostomy ties are to be changed, have an assistant don a sterile glove and hold the tracheostomy tube in place.	
___	___	___	19. Cut a 1/2-inch slit approximately 1 inch from one end of both clean tracheostomy ties. Fold back on itself 1 inch of the tie, and cut a small slit in the middle.	
___	___	___	20. Remove and discard soiled tracheostomy ties.	
___	___	___	21. Thread end of tie through cut slit in tie. Pull tight.	
___	___	___	22. Repeat Steps 19–21 with second tie.	
___	___	___	23. Bring both ties together at one side of client's neck. Assess that ties are only tight enough to allow one finger between tie and neck. Use two square knots to secure the ties. Trim excess tie length. Note: Assess tautness of ties frequently in clients whose neck may swell from trauma or surgery.	
___	___	___	24. Remove gloves and discard disposable equipment. Label with date and time, and store reusable supplies.	
			25. Assist client to comfortable position and offer oral hygiene.	
___	___	___	26. Wash hands and document the procedure and observations.	

Procedure Checklists to Accompany Craven and Hirnle's Fundamentals
of Nursing: Human Health and Function, 5th edition

Name _____   Date _____

Unit _____   Position _____

Instructor/Evaluator: _____   Position _____

Excellent	Satisfactory	Needs Practice	PROCEDURE 36-8 **Suctioning Secretions from Airways**	Comments
			Goal: To maintain patent airway by removing excess secretions, or to collect specimen for diagnostic testing.	
____	____	____	1. Verify physician's order, and identify client.	
____	____	____	2. Wash hands.	
____	____	____	3. Explain procedure and purpose to client.	
____	____	____	4. Position the client.	
____	____	____	a. Position conscious client with an intact gag reflex in semi Fowler's position.	
____	____	____	b. Position the unconscious client in a side-lying position facing you.	
____	____	____	5. Turn suction device on and adjust pressure: infants and children, 50 to 75 mm Hg; adults, 100 to 120 mm Hg.	
____	____	____	6. Open and prepare sterile suction catheter kit.	
____	____	____	a. Unfold sterile cup, touching only the outside. Place on bedside table.	
____	____	____	b. Pour sterile saline into cup.	
____	____	____	7. Preoxygenate client with 100% oxygen. Hyperinflate with manual resuscitation bag.	
____	____	____	8. Don sterile gloves. If kit provides only one glove, place on dominant hand. You may use a clean disposable glove on the nondominant hand to protect yourself from exposure to sputum.	
____	____	____	9. Pick up catheter with dominant hand. Pick up connecting tubing with nondominant hand. Attach catheter to tubing without contaminating sterile hand.	
____	____	____	10. Place catheter end into cup of saline. Test functioning of equipment by applying thumb from nondominant hand over open port to create suction.	
____	____	____	11. Insert catheter into trachea through nostril, nasal trumpet, or artificial airway during inspiration.	
____	____	____	12. Advance catheter until you feel resistance. Retract catheter 1 cm before applying suction. Note: Client usually will cough when catheter enters trachea.	

PROCEDURE 36-8
Suctioning Secretions from Airways (*Continued*)

Goal: To maintain patent airway by removing excess secretions, or to collect specimen for diagnostic testing.

Excellent	Satisfactory	Needs Practice		Comments
____	____	____	13. Apply suction by placing thumb of nondominant hand over open port. Rotate the catheter with your dominant hand as you withdraw the catheter. This should take 5 to 10 seconds.	
____	____	____	14. Hyperoxygenate and hyperinflate using manual resuscitation bag for a full minute between subsequent suction passes. Encourage deep breathing.	
____	____	____	15. Rinse catheter thoroughly with saline.	
____	____	____	16. Repeat Steps 11 to 15 until airway is clear.	
____	____	____	17. Without applying suction, insert the catheter gently along one side of the mouth. Advance to the oropharynx.	
____	____	____	18. Apply suction for 5 to 10 seconds as you rotate and withdraw catheter.	
____	____	____	19. Allow 1 to 2 minutes between passes for the client to ventilate. Encourage deep breathing. Replace oxygen if applicable.	
____	____	____	20. Repeat Steps 17 and 18 as necessary to clear oropharynx.	
____	____	____	21. Rinse catheter and tubing by suctioning saline through.	
____	____	____	22. Remove gloves by holding catheter with dominant hand and pulling glove off inside-out. Catheter will remain coiled inside glove. Pull other glove off inside-out. Dispose of in trash receptacle.	
____	____	____	23. Turn off suction device.	
____	____	____	24. Assist client to comfortable position. Offer assistance with oral and nasal hygiene. Replace oxygen device if used.	
____	____	____	25. Dispose of disposable supplies.	
____	____	____	26. Wash hands	
____	____	____	27. Ensure that sterile suction kit is available at head of bed.	
____	____	____	28. Document procedure and observations.	

Procedure Checklists to Accompany Craven and Hirnle's Fundamentals of Nursing: Human Health and Function, 5th edition

Name _____ Date _____

Unit _____ Position _____

Instructor/Evaluator: _____ Position _____

Excellent	Satisfactory	Needs Practice	PROCEDURE 36-9 **Managing an Obstructed Airway (Heimlich Maneuver)**	Comments
			Goal: To remove a foreign body from obstructing the airway to prevent anoxia and cardiopulmonary arrest.	
			Conscious Child or Adult (Heimlich Maneuver)	
____	____	____	1. Client is standing or sitting.	
____	____	____	2. Stand behind client.	
____	____	____	3. Wrap your arms around client's waist.	
____	____	____	4. Make a fist with one hand. Place thumb side of fist against client's abdomen, above the navel but below the xiphoid process.	
____	____	____	5. Grasp fist with other hand.	
____	____	____	6. Press fist into abdomen with a quick upward thrust.	
____	____	____	7. Repeat distinct separate thrust until the client expels the foreign body or becomes unconscious.	
			Unconscious Client (Heimlich Maneuver, Abdominal Thrust)	
____	____	____	1. Client is lying on ground.	
____	____	____	2. Turn client on back and call for help. Activate emergency response system (911).	
____	____	____	3. Finger sweep: a. Use tongue-jaw lift to open mouth.	
____	____	____	b. Insert index finger inside cheek and sweep to base of tongue. Use hooking motion if possible to dislodge and remove the foreign body. Avoid finger sweeps in infants and children because you can easily push the foreign body further into the airway. Remove only if clearly visible and easy to reach.	
____	____	____	c. If there is no effective breathing, attempt to provide 2 rescue breaths. If unsuccessful, reposition and try to ventilate again.	
____	____	____	4. Straddle client's thighs or kneel to the side of thighs.	
____	____	____	5. Place heel of one hand on epigastric area, midline above the navel but below the xiphoid process.	
____	____	____	6. Place second hand on top of first hand.	

PROCEDURE 36-9
Managing an Obstructed Airway
(Heimlich Maneuver) (*Continued*)

Goal: To remove a foreign body from obstructing the airway to prevent anoxia and cardiopulmonary arrest.

Excellent	Satisfactory	Needs Practice		Comments
___	___	___	7. Press heel of hand into abdomen with a quick upward thrust.	
___	___	___	8. Repeat abdominal thrusts 5 times. Be careful not to thrust in midline to prevent injury to liver or spleen.	
___	___	___	9. If airway is still obstructed, attempt to ventilate using mouth-to-mouth respiration and head tilt/chin lift.	
___	___	___	10. Repeat Steps 5 through 9 until successful.	

Children Younger than One Year of Age (Back Blows and Chest Thrusts)

___	___	___	1. Straddle infant over your arm with head lower than trunk.	
___	___	___	2. Support head by holding jaw firmly in your hand.	
___	___	___	3. Rest your forearm on your thigh and deliver five back blows with the heel of your hand between the infant's scapula.	
___	___	___	4. Place free hand on infant's back and support neck while turning to supine position.	
___	___	___	5. Place two fingers over sternum in same location as for external chest compression (one finger-width below nipple line).	
___	___	___	6. Administer five chest thrusts.	
___	___	___	7. Repeat Steps 1 through 6 until airway is not obstructed.	

Children Older than 1 Year of Age

___	___	___	1. Perform Heimlich maneuver with child standing, sitting, or lying as for adult but more gently.	
___	___	___	2. You may need to kneel behind child or have child stand on a table.	
___	___	___	3. Prevent foreign body airway obstruction in infants and children by teaching parents or caregivers to: a. Restrict children from walking, running, or playing with food or foreign objects in their mouths.	
___	___	___	b. Keep small objects (e.g., marbles, beads, beans, thumb tacks) away from children younger than 3 years.	

PROCEDURE 36-9

Managing an Obstructed Airway (Heimlich Maneuver) (*Continued*)

Excellent	Satisfactory	Needs Practice	

Goal: To remove a foreign body from obstructing the airway to prevent anoxia and cardiopulmonary arrest.

Comments

____ ____ ____   c. Avoid feeding popcorn and peanuts to children younger than 3 years, and cut other foods into small pieces.

____ ____ ____   4. Instruct parents and caregivers in the management of foreign body airway obstruction.

Pregnant Women or Very Obese Adults (Chest Thrusts)

____ ____ ____   1. Stand behind client.

____ ____ ____   2. Bring your arms under client's armpits and around chest.

____ ____ ____   3. Make a fist and place thumb side against middle of sternum.

____ ____ ____   4. Grasp fist with other hand and deliver quick, backward thrust.

____ ____ ____   5. Repeat thrusts until airway is cleared.

____ ____ ____   6. Chest thrusts may be performed with client supine and hands positioned with heel over lower half of sternum. Administer separate, downward thrusts until airway is clear.

Procedure Checklists to Accompany Craven and Hirnle's Fundamentals of Nursing: Human Health and Function, 5th edition

Name _____   Date _____

Unit _____   Position _____

Instructor/Evaluator: _____   Position _____

PROCEDURE 37-1
Applying Antiembolic Stockings

Goal: To supplement the action of muscle contraction to aid venous return from lower extremities and to prevent deep vein thrombosis.

Excellent	Satisfactory	Needs Practice		Comments
____	____	____	1. Position client in supine position for one-half hour before applying stockings.	
____	____	____	2. Provide for the client's privacy, and explain purpose of antiembolic stockings.	
____	____	____	3. Measure for proper fit before first application. Measure length (heel to groin) and width (calf and thigh) and compare to manufacturer's printed material to ensure proper fit.	
____	____	____	4. Make sure legs are dry or apply a light dusting of powder. Turn stocking inside out, tucking the foot inside.	
____	____	____	5. Ease foot section over client's toe and heel, adjusting as necessary for proper smooth fit.	
____	____	____	6. Gently pull stocking over leg, removing all wrinkles.	
____	____	____	7. Assess toes for circulation and warmth. Check area at top of stocking for binding.	
____	____	____	8. Antiembolic stockings should be removed at least twice daily.	

Procedure Checklists to Accompany Craven and Hirnle's Fundamentals
of Nursing: Human Health and Function, 5th edition

Name _____   Date _____

Unit _____   Position _____

Instructor/Evaluator: _____   Position _____

Excellent	Satisfactory	Needs Practice	PROCEDURE 37-2 **Applying a Sequential Compression Device (SCD)** **Goal:** To promote venous return from legs to decrease the risk of deep vein thrombosis and pulmonary embolism in clients with decreased mobility.	Comments
____	____	____	1. Identify client. Explain procedure and purpose to client.	
____	____	____	2. Provide for client's privacy.	
____	____	____	3. Measure leg to ensure proper sleeve sizing.	
____	____	____	a. Knee length: One size fits all.	
____	____	____	b. Thigh length: Measure length of leg from ankle to popliteal fossa. Measure circumference of thigh at the gluteal fold. Use correct sleeve size: Extra small – circumference 22 inches, length 16 inches; Regular – circumference 29 inches, length 16 inches: Extra large – circumference 35 inches, length 16 inches.	
____	____	____	4. Apply antiembolism stockings. Ensure that there are no wrinkles or folds (see Procedure 37-1). Use stockinette or ace wraps if unable to fit client with antiembolism stockings.	
____	____	____	5. Place client in supine position.	
____	____	____	6. Place a plastic sleeve under each leg so the opening is at the knee. If only one sleeve is required, leave the other sleeve in package, and connect to control unit.	
____	____	____	7. Fold outer section of the sleeve over the inner portion, and secure with Velcro tabs. Check sleeve fit. Two fingers should fit between the sleeve and leg.	
____	____	____	8. Connect tubing to control unit. The premarked arrows on the tubing from the sleeve and from the controller must be aligned to make adequate connection. Turn machine on.	
____	____	____	9. Adjust the control unit settings as necessary. Unit control is preset with sleeve cooling in "off" position and audible alarm in "on" position. Sleeve cooling should be in "on" position at all times except during surgery. Ankle pressure should be set at 35 to 55 mm Hg.	
____	____	____	10. Recheck control unit settings whenever unit has been turned off.	

PROCEDURE 37-2

Applying a Sequential Compression Device (SCD) (*Continued*)

Excellent	Satisfactory	Needs Practice		Comments
			Goal: To promote venous return from legs to decrease the risk of deep vein thrombosis and pulmonary embolism in clients with decreased mobility.	
____	____	____	11. Respond to and promptly correct all "fault" indicator alarms. The control unit will sense four pressure "fault" conditions:	
____	____	____	a. Pressure failed to drop to zero during the cycle.	
____	____	____	b. Ankle pressure failed to reach 20 mm Hg.	
____	____	____	c. Ankle pressure exceeded 90 mm Hg.	
			d. Internal diagnostics error has occurred.	
____	____	____	12. Document time and date of application. If SCD is applied to only one leg, document reason.	
			13. Assess and document skin integrity every 8 hours.	
____	____	____	14. Remove sleeves and notify physician if client experiences tingling, numbness, or leg pain.	

Procedure Checklists to Accompany Craven and Hirnle's Fundamentals of Nursing: Human Health and Function, 5th edition

Name _____   Date _____

Unit _____   Position _____

Instructor/Evaluator: _____   Position _____

Excellent	Satisfactory	Needs Practice	PROCEDURE 37-3 **Administering Cardiopulmonary Resuscitation**	Comments
			Goal: To restore cardiopulmonary functioning and prevent irreversible brain damage from anoxia.	
			One Rescuer—Adult Client	
___	___	___	1. Verbally ask "Are you okay?" Assess to determine responsiveness. Shake gently.	
___	___	___	2. Call for help, or activate emergency response system (911).	
___	___	___	3. Turn client onto back while supporting head and neck. Place a cardiac board under the back, or place client on the floor.	
___	___	___	4. Open the airway:	
___	___	___	a. Use the head tilt/chin lift maneuver.	
___	___	___	b. Use the modified jaw thrust if a neck injury is suspected.	
___	___	___	5. Place your ear over client's mouth, and observe the chest for rising with respiration. *Listen, look, and feel* for breathing for 3 to 5 seconds.	
___	___	___	6. Pinch the client's nostrils with thumb and index finger of hand holding the forehead.	
___	___	___	7. Take a deep breath, and place your mouth around the client's mouth with a tight seal. If client wears dentures, they should remain in place.	
___	___	___	8. Ventilate two slow breaths. Each breath should take 2 seconds to deliver. Pause between breaths to allow for lung deflation and to take another deep breath.	
___	___	___	9. If client is breathing but still unresponsive, turn on to side (recovery position).	
___	___	___	10. Assess for carotid pulse for 5 to 10 seconds on the side next to which you are kneeling. Maintain head tilt with the other hand.	
___	___	___	11. If client is pulseless, start chest compressions.	
___	___	___	12. With the hand nearest client's legs, place middle and index fingers on lower ridge or near ribs, and move fingers up along ribs to the costal sternal notch (in center of lower chest).	
___	___	___	13. Place middle finger on this notch and the index finger next to the middle finger on the lower end of the notch.	

PROCEDURE 37-3
Administering Cardiopulmonary Resuscitation (*Continued*)

Excellent	Satisfactory	Needs Practice		Comments
			Goal: To restore cardiopulmonary functioning and prevent irreversible brain damage from anoxia.	
____	____	____	14. Place heel of other hand along the lower half of the sternum, next to the index finger.	
____	____	____	15. Remove first hand from the notch and place heel of that hand parallel over the hand on the chest. Interlock fingers, keeping them off client's chest.	
____	____	____	16. Keeping your hands on sternum, extend your arms, locking the elbows, with your shoulders directly over the client's chest.	
____	____	____	17. Press down on the chest, depressing sternum 1.5 to 2 inches.	
____	____	____	18. Completely release compression while maintaining your hand position. Repeat in a smooth rhythm 100 times/min.	
____	____	____	19. Ventilate with 2 full breaths after every 15 chest compressions.	
____	____	____	20. Repeat 4 cycles of 15 chest compressions and 2 ventilations.	
____	____	____	21. Reassess for carotid pulse. If client is pulseless, continue CPR. Reassess for carotid pulse every few minutes without interrupting CPR for more than 7 seconds.	

Two Rescuers—Adult Client

____	____	____	1. When second rescuer arrives, the first rescuer stops CPR after completing two ventilations and assesses for a carotid pulse for 5 seconds.	
____	____	____	2. The second rescuer moves into the chest compression position.	
____	____	____	3. If pulselessness continues, the first rescuer states "no pulse" and delivers one ventilation.	
____	____	____	4. The second rescuer begins chest compression while counting out loud, "one and two and three and four and five and. . ." The compression rate is 100/min.	
____	____	____	5. The first rescuer gives two slow ventilations after 15 chest compressions. The first rescuer also assesses carotid pulse during chest compressions to evaluate effectiveness.	
____	____	____	6. If second rescuer wishes to change positions, he or she states, "Change, one and two and three and four and five and. . ."	
____	____	____	7. The first rescuer delivers the ventilation then moves into the chest compression position.	

Excellent	Satisfactory	Needs Practice	PROCEDURE 37-3 ## Administering Cardiopulmonary ## Resuscitation (*Continued*)	Comments
			Goal: To restore cardiopulmonary functioning and prevent irreversible brain damage from anoxia.	
——	——	——	8. The second rescuer moves to the ventilator position and assesses for a carotid pulse for 5 seconds. If pulseless, resume CPR. Do not interrupt CPR for more than 7 seconds.	
			One Rescuer CPR—Infant and Child	
——	——	——	1. Assess unresponsiveness.	
——	——	——	2. If unresponsive, activate emergency response system (911) for children older than 8 years.	
——	——	——	3. Place child on hard surface. For children older than 8 years of age, provide basic life support for 1 full minute before activating emergency medical system.	
——	——	——	4. Open the airway using the head tilt/chin lift. Avoid overextension of head in infants.	
——	——	——	5. Place your ear over child's mouth, and observe chest for rise. Listen, look, and feel for breathing. Perform Heimlich maneuver if airway obstruction from food or foreign object is suspected. Procedure 36-9.	
——	——	——	6. If breathlessness is determined, seal mouth and nose and ventilate twice (1–1.5 seconds for each breath). Observe for chest rise. In infants and small children, rescuer may need to place mouth over the mouth and nose to establish an airtight seal.	
——	——	——	7. Assess pulselessness by palpating for carotid artery on near side in children older than 1 year. In infants younger than 1 year, assess brachial or femoral pulse for 5 seconds.	
——	——	——	8. Begin chest compression if pulseless.	
——	——	——	a. For infant up to 1 year:	
——	——	——	(1) Visualize an imaginary line between the infant's nipples.	
——	——	——	(2) Place your index finger on the sternum just below this imaginary line.	
——	——	——	(3) Place your middle and fourth finger on sternum next to index finger.	
——	——	——	b. For child 1 to 8 years of age:	
——	——	——	(1) Placement of hand on sternum is the same as for adult CPR. Use heel of one hand to compress sternum 1 to 1½ inches 100 times/min.	
——	——	——	(2) Continue chest compressions, and ventilate at the rate of one breath to five compressions.	
——	——	——	(3) Continue CPR as for an adult.	

*Procedure Checklists to Accompany Craven and Hirnle's Fundamentals
of Nursing: Human Health and Function,* 5th edition

Name _____ Date _____

Unit _____ Position _____

Instructor/Evaluator: _____ Position _____

Excellent	Satisfactory	Needs Practice	PROCEDURE 39-1 **Measuring Blood Glucose by Skin Puncture**	Comments
			Goal: To monitor blood glucose levels for clients who are at risk for hypoglycemia or hyperglycemia, and to monitor effectiveness of insulin administration.	
____	____	____	1. Have client wash hands with soap and warm water.	
____	____	____	2. Position client comfortably.	
____	____	____	3. Remove reagent strip from the container and handle according to the manufacturer's instructions.	
____	____	____	4. Place reagent strip with test pad up on a dry surface.	
____	____	____	5. Choose the finger to be punctured, massage gently, and hold in a dependent position.	
____	____	____	6. If part of agency's procedure, wipe the puncture site with alcohol. Allow site to dry completely.	
____	____	____	7. Don gloves.	
____	____	____	8. Remove the cover of the lancet or autolet. Place the autolet against the side of the finger and push the release button. If using a lancet, hold it perpendicular to the site, and pierce the site quickly.	
____	____	____	9. Wipe the initial drop of blood with a cotton ball.	
____	____	____	10. Squeeze the puncture gently or massage the skin toward the site to obtain a large drop of blood. Hold reagent strip next to drop of blood, and allow blood to cover the test pad completely. Do not smear the blood. In some meters, bring the finger to the test site on the meter, and allow blood to drop onto appropriate area.	
____	____	____	11. Start timing (usually less than 60 seconds) using the glucose meter or a watch if the meter is not available.	
____	____	____	12. Following manufacturer's instruction, wipe the blood from the test pad with a cotton ball after the specified period of time. Note: Slight variations may occur in the procedure between different manufacturers.	

PROCEDURE 39-1

Measuring Blood Glucose by Skin Puncture (*Continued*)

Goal: To monitor blood glucose levels for clients who are at risk for hypoglycemia or hyperglycemia, and to monitor effectiveness of insulin administration.

Excellent	Satisfactory	Needs Practice		Comments
____	____	____	13. Place the reagent strip into the glucose meter. After the recommended period of time, read the results. For meters on which blood is placed directly, read the results at the designated time. If a glucose meter is not available, compare the color of the test pad with the color strip on the side of the reagent strip container.	
____	____	____	14. Turn off the glucose meter. Dispose of used equipment in the appropriate manner (needles in used needle receptacle).	
____	____	____	15. Share test results with client, and record obtained values in the client's chart.	

Procedure Checklists to Accompany Craven and Hirnle's Fundamentals of Nursing: Human Health and Function, 5th edition

Name _____   Date _____

Unit _____   Position _____

Instructor/Evaluator: _____   Position _____

Excellent	Satisfactory	Needs Practice	PROCEDURE 39-2 **Assisting an Adult with Feeding**	Comments
			Goal: To maintain nutritional status.	
___	___	___	1. Prepare client's environment for meal:	
___	___	___	a. Remove urinals, bedpans, dressings, and trash.	
___	___	___	b. Ventilate or aerate room for unpleasant odors.	
___	___	___	c. Clean overbed table.	
___	___	___	2. Prepare client for meal:	
___	___	___	a. Help client to urinate or defecate.	
___	___	___	b. Help client to wash face and hands.	
___	___	___	c. Assist with oral hygiene.	
___	___	___	d. Help client to apply dentures, glasses, or special appliances.	
___	___	___	e. Assist to upright position in bed or chair.	
___	___	___	3. Wash your hands before touching meal tray.	
___	___	___	4. Check client's tray against diet order and with client's identification.	
___	___	___	5. Place tray on overbed table and move in front of client.	
___	___	___	6. Prepare tray. Open cartons, remove lids, season food, and cut food into bite-size pieces.	
___	___	___	7. Place napkin or towel under client's chin, and cover clothing.	
___	___	___	8. If client can feed self, leave and return in 10 to 15 minutes to determine if client is tolerating diet. (Do not leave client with overly hot liquids or food unless fully independent with feeding.)	
___	___	___	9. a. If client can sit in a chair but needs help to eat, sit in chair facing client.	
___	___	___	b. If client must remain in bed, you may stand to feed client.	
___	___	___	10. Allow client to choose the order in which he or she would like to eat. If client is visually impaired, identify the food on the tray.	
___	___	___	11. Warn client if food is hot or cold.	
___	___	___	12. Allow enough time between bites for adequate chewing and swallowing.	
___	___	___	13. Offer liquids as requested or between bites. Use straw or special drinking cup if available.	

Excellent	Satisfactory	Needs Practice	PROCEDURE 39-2 **Assisting an Adult with Feeding (*Continued*)**
			Goal: To maintain nutritional status. **Comments**
____ ____ ____			14. Provide conversation during meal. Choose topic of interest to client. Reorient to current events or use meal as opportunity to educate on nutrition or discharge plans. Note: Do **not** talk to clients who are relearning swallowing techniques; they need to concentrate.
____ ____ ____			15. Help client to wash hands and face, and perform oral hygiene after meal.
____ ____ ____			16. Assist to comfortable position and allow rest period. If at risk for aspiration, leave head of bed elevated for 30 minutes after eating.
____ ____ ____			17. Record fluids and amount of meal consumed, if ordered.
____ ____ ____			18. Remove and dispose of tray.
____ ____ ____			19. Wash hands.

Procedure Checklists to Accompany Craven and Hirnle's Fundamentals
of Nursing: Human Health and Function, 5th edition

Name _____   Date _____

Unit _____   Position _____

Instructor/Evaluator: _____   Position _____

PROCEDURE 39-3
Administering Nutrition via Nasogastric or Gastrostomy Tube

Goal: To provide enteral nutrition for clients who cannot swallow or have an esophageal obstruction, or who are comatose or semiconscious, or who cannot consume adequate calories orally.

Excellent	Satisfactory	Needs Practice		Comments

1. Wash hands.
2. Close room door or curtains around bed.
3. Explain procedure to client.
4. Help client to high Fowler's position by moving client up to the head of the bed, then elevating head of bed at least 60 degrees or assisting to chair. If high Fowler's position is contraindicated, help client to a right side-lying position with head slightly elevated.
5. Confirm placement of tube in stomach:
   a. Withdraw sample of stomach contents, and check for low pH level.
   b. Attach 60 mL irrigation syringe to tube, and inject 10 mL of air while auscultating over epigastrium. Recognize that this may not be reliable index of tube placement when client has small-bore feeding tube.
   c. Aspirate all stomach contents, and measure for residual.
   d. If 100 mL or more than half of last feeding is aspirated, contact physician before proceeding with tube feeding. The feeding is usually held.
   e. Reinstill the aspirated gastric contents through tube into stomach.
6. Prepare correct amount and strength of formula at room temperature. (Optional: Add several drops of food coloring.)

Bolus of Intermittent Feeding

1. Remove plunger from irrigation syringe. Clamp gastric tubing and attach syringe. If using gavage bag, attach tubing to gastric tube.
2. Fill syringe or gavage bag with formula.

Excellent	Satisfactory	Needs Practice	PROCEDURE 39-3 **Administering Nutrition via Nasogastric or Gastrostomy Tube (*Continued*)**	
			Goal: To provide enteral nutrition for clients who cannot swallow or have an esophageal obstruction, or who are comatose or semiconscious, or who cannot consume adequate calories orally.	**Comments**
——	——	——	3. Allow feeding to flow in slowly over 10 to 15 minutes. If using syringe, raise and lower to adjust flow rate by gravity. Refill syringe as needed without disconnecting, avoiding air spaces in tubing. If gavage bag is used, hang bag on IV pole, and adjust flow rate with clamp on tubing.	
——	——	——	4. Clamp tubing just as feeding is completing. Rinse tube with 30 to 60 mL tap water. Do **not** allow air to enter tubing.	
——	——	——	5. Clamp gastric tube, and disconnect from syringe or gavage bag.	
——	——	——	6. Have client remain in high Fowler's or elevated side-lying position for 30 to 60 minutes.	
			Continuous Feeding	
——	——	——	1. Connect gavage tubing to gastric tube.	
——	——	——	2. Hang gavage bag on IV pole.	
——	——	——	3. Pour in desired amount of formula according to agency policy (usually amount to infuse in 3 hours).	
——	——	——	4. a. Connect tubing to infusion pump.	
——	——	——	b. Set rate.	
——	——	——	5. Check residual every 4 to 6 hours, according to agency policy. Then flush tubing with 30 to 60 mL water.	
——	——	——	6. Have client remain in high Fowler's or slightly elevated side-lying position.	
——	——	——	7. Wash any reusable equipment with soap and water. Change equipment every 24 hours or according to agency policy.	
——	——	——	8. Wash hands.	
——	——	——	9. Document procedure and observations.	

Procedure Checklists to Accompany Craven and Hirnle's Fundamentals of Nursing: Human Health and Function, 5th edition

Name _____   Date _____

Unit _____   Position _____

Instructor/Evaluator: _____   Position _____

Excellent	Satisfactory	Needs Practice	PROCEDURE 40-1 **Changing a Dry Sterile Dressing**	Comments
			Goal: To protect wound from trauma and external contamination and to provide an opportunity to assess wound.	
____	____	____	1. Close client's door or close curtains around bed. Explain procedure to client.	
____	____	____	2. Position client comfortably. Expose only wound area.	
____	____	____	3. Wash hands.	
____	____	____	4. Make a cuff on top of plastic bag, and place within easy reach of dressing table.	
____	____	____	5. Put on clean disposable gloves.	
____	____	____	6. Remove dressing from wound, and discard into plastic bag. If dressing adheres to wound, pour small amount of sterile saline on wound to loosen dressing.	
____	____	____	7. Remove and dispose of gloves. Wash hands.	
____	____	____	8. Set up sterile supplies:	
____	____	____	a. Open sterile towel, and hold it by edges.	
____	____	____	b. Place it on clean, flat surface without contaminating center of towel.	
____	____	____	c. Open dressing package(s) by peeling paper down to expose dressing. Let it fall onto sterile field.	
____	____	____	d. Open cleansing solution container, and pour solution into sterile cup.	
____	____	____	e. Open any supplies for wound irrigation, and set materials at side of sterile field. (Alternatively, open dressing packages and suture set carefully, allowing the inside of the packaging material to serve as the sterile field.)	
____	____	____	9. Don sterile gloves. Grasp applicators at nonabsorbent end, and dip into cleansing solution.	
____	____	____	10. Clean drainage from center of wound outward, using each applicator only once and discarding without placing applicator back into cleansing solution.	
____	____	____	11. Dry surrounding skin gently with gauze.	
____	____	____	12. Inspect incision for bleeding, inflammation, drainage, and healing. Note any areas of dehiscence.	
____	____	____	13. Apply sterile dressings one at a time over wound.	
____	____	____	14. Wash hands.	
____	____	____	15. Document procedure and observations.	

Procedure Checklists to Accompany Craven and Hirnle's Fundamentals of Nursing: Human Health and Function, 5th edition

Name _____ Date _____

Unit _____ Position _____

Instructor/Evaluator: _____ Position _____

Excellent	Satisfactory	Needs Practice	PROCEDURE 40-2 **Applying Saline-Moistened Dressings**	Comments
			Goal: To promote moist wound healing.	
____	____	____	1. Prepare client and remove dressing according to Steps 1 through 5 of Procedure 40-1. Forceps may be used to remove soiled dressing. If dressing adheres to underlying tissues, moisten with saline to loosen. Gently remove the dressing while assessing client's discomfort level.	
____	____	____	2. Observe dressings for amount and characteristics of drainage. Note odor and color.	
____	____	____	3. Observe wound for eschar, granulation tissue, or epithelial skin buds. Measure and record wound depth, diameter, and length.	
____	____	____	4. Prepare sterile supplies. Open sterile instruments, sterile basin, solution, and dressings.	
____	____	____	5. Place fine-mesh gauze into basin, and pour the ordered solution over mesh to saturate. For large wounds, warm ordered solution to body temperature.	
____	____	____	6. Don sterile gloves.	
____	____	____	7. Cleanse or irrigate wound as prescribed or with normal saline, moving from least to most contaminated areas.	
____	____	____	8. Squeeze excess fluid from gauze dressing. Unfold and fluff out the dressing.	
____	____	____	a. Gently pack moistened gauze into the wound.	
____	____	____	b. If wound is deep, use forceps or cotton-tipped applicators to press gauze into all wound surfaces.	
____	____	____	9. Apply several dry, sterile 4×4s over the wet gauze.	
____	____	____	10. Place ABD pad over dry 4×4s.	
____	____	____	11. Remove and dispose of sterile gloves.	
____	____	____	12. Secure dressings with tape, Kerlix gauze, or Montgomery ties.	
____	____	____	13. Assist client to a comfortable position.	
____	____	____	14. Wash hands.	
____	____	____	15. Document the procedure and observations.	

Procedure Checklists to Accompany Craven and Hirnle's Fundamentals of Nursing: Human Health and Function, 5th edition

Name _____ Date _____

Unit _____ Position _____

Instructor/Evaluator: _____ Position _____

PROCEDURE 40-3
Irrigating a Wound

Goal: To cleanse wound by removing debris and exudate and promote wound healing.

Excellent	Satisfactory	Needs Practice		Comments
____	____	____	1. Close door or curtains around bed. Explain procedure to client.	
____	____	____	2. Position client comfortably to allow irrigating solution to flow by gravity across wound and into a collection basin.	
____	____	____	3. Expose the wound area only. Place waterproof pad under client.	
____	____	____	4. Wash hands.	
____	____	____	5. Don mask, goggles, and gown if needed.	
____	____	____	6. Remove dressing and inspect wound. See Steps 1 through 4 of Procedure 40-2.	
____	____	____	7. Pour warmed irrigating solution into sterile basin.	
____	____	____	8. Open irrigating syringe, and place into basin with solution.	
____	____	____	9. Place second basin at distal end of wound to catch contaminated irrigating solution.	
____	____	____	10. Don sterile gloves.	
____	____	____	11. Fill irrigating syringe with solution. Holding syringe tip about 1 inch above the wound, gently flush all areas of wound. Continue flushing until solution draining into basin is clear.	
____	____	____	12. If wound is deep, attach latex or silicone catheter to syringe filled with irrigating solution. Gently insert catheter into wound and flush until returning solution is clear.	
____	____	____	13. Dry surrounding skin thoroughly.	
____	____	____	14. Apply sterile dressing.	
____	____	____	15. Remove and discard gloves.	
____	____	____	16. Secure dressing with tape or Montgomery straps.	
____	____	____	17. Assist client to comfortable position.	
____	____	____	18. Dispose of equipment. Retain remaining bottle of sterile solution for future irrigations. Mark date and time of opening on bottle for reference. Dispose according to agency policy.	
____	____	____	19. Wash hands.	
____	____	____	20. Document procedure and observations.	

Procedure Checklists to Accompany Craven and Hirnle's Fundamentals of Nursing: Human Health and Function, 5th edition

Name _____   Date _____

Unit _____   Position _____

Instructor/Evaluator: _____   Position _____

Excellent	Satisfactory	Needs Practice	PROCEDURE 40-4 **Maintaining a Portable (HEMOVAC) Wound Suction**	
			Goal: To facilitate healing by removing drainage from the incisional area.	**Comments**
____	____	____	1. Explain procedure, assist client to comfortable position, and pull curtains or close door.	
____	____	____	2. Wash hands. Don clean, disposable gloves.	
____	____	____	3. Expose Hemovac tubing and container while keeping client draped.	
____	____	____	4. Examine tubing and container for patency and suction seal.	
____	____	____	5. Open drainage plug.	
____	____	____	6. Pour drainage into a calibrated receptacle without contaminating drainage spout.	
____	____	____	7. Reestablish suction by placing reservoir on firm, flat surface. With drainage plug open, compress the unit and reinsert drainage plug.	
____	____	____	8. Remove and discard gloves.	
____	____	____	9. Return client to comfortable position.	
____	____	____	10. Measure drainage, and record amount, color, and other pertinent information.	

Procedure Checklists to Accompany Craven and Hirnle's Fundamentals of Nursing: Human Health and Function, 5th edition

Name _____ Date _____

Unit _____ Position _____

Instructor/Evaluator: _____ Position _____

PROCEDURE 41-1
Obtaining a Wound Culture

Goal: To identify organisms colonized within a wound so antibiotics sensitive to the microorganisms can be prescribed as needed.

Excellent	Satisfactory	Needs Practice		Comments
____	____	____	1. Identify client, and verify order for culture, noting site and type of culture.	
____	____	____	2. Wash hands, and apply clean disposable gloves.	
____	____	____	3. Remove soiled dressing. Observe drainage for amount, odor, and color.	
____	____	____	4. Clear and remove exudate from around wound with antiseptic swab.	
			Obtaining Aerobic Culture	
____	____	____	1. Perform Steps 1 to 4 above.	
____	____	____	2. Using sterile swab from culture tube, insert swab deep into area of active drainage. Rotate swab to absorb as much drainage as possible.	
____	____	____	3. Insert swab into culture tube, taking care not to touch the top or outside of tube.	
____	____	____	4. Crush ampule of medium, and close container securely.	
____	____	____	5. Continue with Step 4 below.	
			Obtaining Anaerobic Culture	
____	____	____	1. Perform Steps 1 to 4 at beginning of procedure.	
____	____	____	2. Using sterile swab from special anaerobic culture tube, insert swab deeply into draining body cavity.	
____	____	____	3. a. Rotate swab gently and remove. Quickly place swab into inner tube of collection container.	
____	____	____	b. *Alternative method*: Insert tip of syringe with needle removed into wound and aspirate 1 to 5 mL of exudate. Attach 21-gauge needle to syringe, expel all air, and inject exudate into inner tube of the culture container. Note: Drainage is sample from only one drainage site per culture swab. Repeat above steps for other drainage sites.	
____	____	____	4. Label each culture tube, and send specimens with appropriate requisitions to the laboratory according to agency policy.	

PROCEDURE 41-1
Obtaining a Wound Culture (*Continued*)

Goal: To identify organisms colonized within a wound so antibiotics sensitive to the microorganisms can be prescribed as needed.

Excellent	Satisfactory	Needs Practice		Comments
____	____	____	5. Clean and apply sterile dressings to the wound as ordered.	
____	____	____	6. Remove and discard gloves. Wash hands.	
____	____	____	7. Assist client to comfortable position.	
____	____	____	8. Document all relevant information on client's chart. Include the location from which the specimen was taken and the date and time. Record the wound's consistency of drainage. Record how the client tolerated the procedure and any discomfort from the experience.	

Procedure Checklists to Accompany Craven and Hirnle's Fundamentals of Nursing: Human Health and Function, 5th edition

Name _____   Date _____

Unit _____   Position _____

Instructor/Evaluator: _____   Position _____

PROCEDURE 42-1
Assessing Urine Volume Using a Bladder Ultrasonic Scanner

Goal: To noninvasively calculate the volume of urine in the bladder and to determine the need for catheterization to relieve urinary retention.

Excellent	Satisfactory	Needs Practice		Comments
____	____	____	1. Identify the client and explain the procedure.	
____	____	____	2. Wash hands. Put on disposable gloves.	
____	____	____	3. Provide privacy. Expose only the client's lower abdomen and suprapubic area.	
____	____	____	4. Assist the client to lie as flat as can be comfortably tolerated.	
____	____	____	5. Clean off scanhead probe (soundwave transducer) with isopropyl alcohol.	
____	____	____	6. Turn the bladder scan on and press "SCAN."	
____	____	____	7. Apply ultrasonic gel to scanhead.	
____	____	____	8. Press "MALE" or "FEMALE" mode on scan device. If a female client has had a hysterectomy (removal of uterus), press MALE.	
____	____	____	9. Find the symphysis pubis (midline below the umbilicus) and place the scanhead approximately 3 cm. superior to the symphysis pubis pointing toward the expected bladder location. Locate the icon on the scanhead and point the icon toward the head of the client.	
____	____	____	10. Press the scanhead button and hold the scanhead steady until a beep is heard, then release.	
____	____	____	11. The bladder scan will display the bladder volume measurement and an aiming display. Adjust scanhead aim to obtain intersection of the cross hair and the bladder. Reposition the scanhead and repeat the measurement as needed to obtain a centered image.	
____	____	____	12. When finished, press "DONE."	
____	____	____	13. Press "PRINT" for a hard copy of results.	
____	____	____	14. Wipe gel from client's skin and reposition client if needed.	
____	____	____	15. Dispose of contaminated supplies. Clean scanhead with isopropyl alcohol. Wash hands.	
____	____	____	16. Document procedure and observations.	

*Procedure Checklists to Accompany Craven and Hirnle's Fundamentals
of Nursing: Human Health and Function,* 5th edition

Name _____   Date _____

Unit _____   Position _____

Instructor/Evaluator: _____   Position _____

Excellent	Satisfactory	Needs Practice	PROCEDURE 42-2 ## Collecting Urine Specimens **Goal:** To obtain a noncontaminated urine specimen for routine analysis or culture and sensitivity.	Comments
			Collecting Sterile Specimen From an Indwelling Catheter	
____	____	____	1. Confirm physician's order, and identify client using two separate identifiers (name, medical record number or birthdate).	
____	____	____	2. Explain procedure to client.	
____	____	____	3. Wash hands. Put on disposable gloves.	
____	____	____	4. Position client so that catheter is accessible.	
____	____	____	5. Drain urine from tubing into collection bag. Allow fresh urine to collect in tubing by clamping or bending tubing (2 mL of urine is sufficient for a culture and sensitivity specimen; 30 mL for urinalysis).	
____	____	____	6. Cleanse aspiration port of drainage tubing with alcohol or povidone-iodine (Betadine) swab.	
____	____	____	7. Insert syringe into aspiration port. Draw urine sample into syringe by gentle aspiration. Remove needle.	
____	____	____	8. Transfer urine from syringe into a sterile specimen container. Agency policy may allow transport of specimen to laboratory in syringe with sterile cap in place of needle.	
____	____	____	9. Identify client with at least 2 identifiers (name, medical record number, birthdate) and match this information to label on container. Date and time on laboratory requisition. Place in plastic biohazard bag for delivery to laboratory.	
____	____	____	10. Send specimen to laboratory within 15 minutes, or place in specimen refrigerator. If specimen is for microbiology testing, do **not** refrigerate; send immediately.	
____	____	____	11. Dispose of all contaminated supplies. Wash hands.	
____	____	____	12. Document procedure and observations.	

Excellent	Satisfactory	Needs Practice	

PROCEDURE 42-2
Collecting Urine Specimens (*Continued*)

Goal: To obtain a noncontaminated urine specimen for routine analysis or culture and sensitivity.

Comments

Self-Collecting Midstream Urine Specimen for a Woman

1. Instruct client how to cleanse urinary meatus and obtain urine specimen.
   a. (Client) Wash hands.
   b. Separate labia minora and cleanse perineum with commercially prepared aseptic swabs, starting in front of the urethral meatus and moving swab toward the rectum.
   c. Repeat cleansing process 3 times with different cotton balls or swabs.
   d. Begin to urinate while continuing to hold labia apart. Allow first urine to flow into toilet.
   e. Hold specimen container under the urine stream and collect sample.
   f. Remove specimen container, release hand from labia, seal container tightly, and finish voiding. Wash hands.

2. (Nurse) Put on disposable gloves to receive specimen container from the client. Dry outside of container with a paper towel.

3. Date and time on laboratory specimen. Verify client by 2 identifiers and make sure they match the label. Label the container, and place specimen container in biohazard bag.

4. Send specimen to laboratory within 15 minutes, or place in specimen refrigerator. If specimen is for microbiology testing, do **not** refrigerate; send immediately.

5. Dispose of all contaminated supplies. Wash hands. Multiplying bacteria may split urea, producintg a more alcoholic urine.

Self-Collecting Midstream Urine Specimen for a Man

1. Confirm physician's order, and identify client with at least 2 identifiers.

2. Instruct client how to cleanse urinary meatus and obtain urine specimen.
   a. (Client) Wash hands.
   b. Starting at top in a circular motion, cleanse end of penis with cotton balls and soap or commercially prepared antiseptic swab. If man is not circumcised, instruct him to retract foreskin

Excellent	Satisfactory	Needs Practice	PROCEDURE 42-2 **Collecting Urine Specimens (*Continued*)**	Comments
			Goal: To obtain a noncontaminated urine specimen for routine analysis or culture and sensitivity.	

___ ___ ___		to expose urinary meatus before cleansing and throughout specimen collection.
___ ___ ___		c. Repeat cleansing three times with 3 separate cotton balls or aseptic swabs.
___ ___ ___		d. Begin to urinate, allowing urine to flow into toilet.
___ ___ ___		e. Pass specimen container into urine stream and collect sample.
___ ___ ___		f. Remove container, seal tightly, and finish voiding.
		3. Follow Steps 2 to 5 above.

Collecting a Specimen From a Child Without Urinary Control

___ ___ ___	1. Confirm physician's order and identify client using at least 2 identifiers.
___ ___ ___	2. If parents are present, explain procedure to them.
___ ___ ___	3. Position child gently on back. Put on disposable gloves. Remove diaper.
	4. Clean perineal-genital area gently with soap and water, followed by antiseptic.
___ ___ ___	5. For a girl: Separate labia and cleanse from front of urethral meatus toward rectum. Rinse with water and dry with cotton balls.
	6. For a boy: Cleanse penis and scrotum. If uncircumcised, retract foreskin and cleanse. Rinse with water and dry with gauze or cotton balls.
___ ___ ___	7. Remove paper backing from adhesive of collection bag.
___ ___ ___	8. Spread child's legs apart widely.
___ ___ ___	9. Apply collection bag over child's perineum, covering penis and scrotum of boy and urinary meatus and vagina of girl. Press adhesive to secure, starting at perineum and working outward.
___ ___ ___	10. Place a diaper on child loosely.
___ ___ ___	11. Remove gloves and wash hands.
___ ___ ___	12. Check the collector for urine every 15 minutes. Parents can be instructed to check child for urine specimen.
___ ___ ___	13. When urine specimen is obtained, glove again, and gently remove collection bag from skin, and empty urine into specimen container.

PROCEDURE 42-2
Collecting Urine Specimens (*Continued*)

Goal: To obtain a noncontaminated urine specimen for routine analysis or culture and sensitivity.

Excellent	Satisfactory	Needs Practice		Comments
____	____	____	14. Tighten lid and cleanse outside of container if contaminated with urine, and place in plastic biohazard bag for transfer to laboratory.	
____	____	____	15. Label the container making sure that it is correct client information. Record date and time on laboratory requisition.	
____	____	____	16. Send specimen to laboratory within 15 minutes, or place in specimen refrigerator. If specimen is for microbiology testing, do **not** refrigerate; send immediately. Send immediately if specimen is for microbiology testing; do **not** refrigerate.	
____	____	____	17. Dispose of all contaminated supplies. Wash hands.	
____	____	____	18. Document that specimen was collected and sent.	

Procedure Checklists to Accompany Craven and Hirnle's Fundamentals of Nursing: Human Health and Function, 5th edition

Name _____ Date _____

Unit _____ Position _____

Instructor/Evaluator: _____ Position _____

PROCEDURE 42-3
Applying a Condom Catheter

Goal: To provide a means of collecting urine and controlling incontinence without the risk of infection that an indwelling urinary catheter imposes.

Excellent	Satisfactory	Needs Practice		Comments
____	____	____	1. Close room door or bedside curtain. Explain procedure to client.	
____	____	____	2. Wash hands.	
____	____	____	3. Assist client to supine position with only genitalia exposed.	
____	____	____	4. Put on disposable gloves. Wash client's genitals with soap and water. Towel dry. For uncircumcised male, be sure that foreskin is not retracted.	
____	____	____	5. Trim excess pubic hair from base of penis, if necessary.	
____	____	____	6. Apply thin film of skin protector on penis shaft. (Skin protector usually found in commercially packaged condom catheter kits.). Allow to dry for 30 seconds.	
____	____	____	7. Peel paper backing from both sides of adhesive liner and wrap spirally around penis shaft.	
____	____	____	8. Place funnel end of pre-rolled condom against glans of penis. Unroll sheath the length of the penis, over the adhesive liner. Some brands of condom catheters are held in place with a Velcro strap over the condom catheter.	
____	____	____	9. Attach funnel end of condom to collection system. Tape may be used to secure the connection below level of condom, avoiding kinks or loops in tubing.	
____	____	____	10. Discard used supplies and wash hands.	
____	____	____	11. Observe penis 15 to 30 minutes after application of condom for swelling or changes in skin color. (If too tight, remove and reapply larger size.)	
____	____	____	12. Document procedure and observations.	

Procedure Checklists to Accompany Craven and Hirnle's Fundamentals of Nursing: Human Health and Function, 5th edition

Name _____   Date _____

Unit _____   Position _____

Instructor/Evaluator: _____   Position _____

Excellent	Satisfactory	Needs Practice	PROCEDURE 42-4 **Inserting a Straight or Indwelling Urinary Catheter**	
			Goal: To monitor urinary function, relieve bladder distension, provide continuous bladder drainage, obtain sterile urine specimen, or provide a means for irrigating the bladder.	**Comments**
____	____	____	1. Verify physician's order, and identify the client.	
____	____	____	2. Explain procedure and rationale to client.	
____	____	____	3. Provide client with opportunity to perform personal perineal/penile hygiene. Assist client as necessary.	
____	____	____	4. Wash your hands.	
			Inserting Catheter for a Woman	
____	____	____	1. Position in dorsal recumbent position. Externally rotate thighs. Side-lying is alternate position.	
____	____	____	2. Set up light source.	
____	____	____	3. Open catheterization tray, maintaining asepsis.	
____	____	____	4. Slide sterile drape under client's buttocks, grasping corners of drape. Ask client to lift hips so drape can be slid under.	
____	____	____	5. Don sterile gloves.	
____	____	____	6. Open sterile lubricant, and lubricate catheter tip. Open cleansing solution, and pour over half of the sterile cotton balls. Open sterile specimen container. Inflate balloon with prefilled syringe to check for defective balloon. Aspirate fluid back into syringe and leave attached.	
____	____	____	7. Place nondominant hand on labia minora and gently spread to expose urinary meatus. Visualize exact location of meatus. During cleansing and catheter insertion, do **not** allow labia to close over meatus until after catheter is inserted.	
____	____	____	8. Using sterile hand, pick up antiseptic solution-saturated cotton ball with sterile forceps.	
____	____	____	9. Cleanse urinary meatus with one downward stroke. Discard cotton ball. Repeat this step three or four times.	
____	____	____	10. Use forceps and dry cotton balls to absorb excess antiseptic solution.	

PROCEDURE 42-4
Inserting a Straight or Indwelling Urinary Catheter (*Continued*)

Goal: To monitor urinary function, relieve bladder distension, provide continuous bladder drainage, obtain sterile urine specimen, or provide a means for irrigating the bladder.

Excellent	Satisfactory	Needs Practice		Comments
____	____	____	11. With sterile hand, pick up catheter approximately 3 inch from tip and dip into sterile lubricant (2% Lidocaine gel may be used). Place distal catheter end into sterile basin.	
____	____	____	12. Gently insert catheter into urethra approximately 2 inch until urine begins to drain. If no urine appears, have client cough, or reposition catheter by rotating. Have client take slow, deep breaths during catheter insertion.	
____	____	____	13. Insert catheter an additional 1 inch (2.5 cm). If catheter enters vagina by mistake, leave it there as a landmark. Insert second catheter into meatus.	
____	____	____	14. Obtain urine specimen in sterile container, if ordered.	
____	____	____	15. If using straight catheter: Allow bladder to empty, then remove straight catheter. Measure urine volume.	
____	____	____	16. If using indwelling catheter: Inflate the retention balloon with the prefilled syringe. Check to ensure placement by gently pulling on catheter.	
____	____	____	17. Connect distal end of catheter to drainage bag (may prefer to connect prior to catheter insertion). In some kits, the catheter is already connected to the drainage unit.	
____	____	____	18. Tape catheter securely with 1-inch tape to inner thigh with enough give so it will not pull when moving the legs.	
____	____	____	19. Attach drainage bag to bed frame, ensuring that tubing does not fall into dependent loops or that side rails do not interfere with drainage system.	
____	____	____	20. Remove gloves. Wash hands.	
____	____	____	21. Record time of completion of procedure, size of catheter inserted, amount and color of urine, and any adverse client responses.	

Inserting Catheter for a Man

Excellent	Satisfactory	Needs Practice		Comments
____	____	____	1. Position client in supine position with only genitalia exposed.	
____	____	____	2. Drape legs to mid-thigh with bath blanket or sheet.	
____	____	____	3. Open catheterization tray.	

PROCEDURE 42-4
Inserting a Straight or Indwelling Urinary Catheter (*Continued*)

Excellent	**Satisfactory**	**Needs Practice**	**Goal:** To monitor urinary function, relieve bladder distension, provide continuous bladder drainage, obtain sterile urine specimen, or provide a means for irrigating the bladder.	**Comments**

Excellent	Satisfactory	Needs Practice		Comments
___	___	___	4. Put on sterile gloves. Open sterile lubricant and lubricate catheter tip. Open cleansing solution and pour over half of the sterile cotton balls. Open sterile specimen container. Inflate balloon with prefilled syringe to check for defective balloon. Aspirate fluid back into syringe and leave attached.	
___	___	___	5. Place the fenestrated drape over the client's genitalia.	
___	___	___	6. With nondominant hand, hold penis at a 90-degree angle to his body. If client is not circumcised, pull back foreskin with this hand to visualize the urethral meatus.	
___	___	___	7. Using the sterile hand, pick up antiseptic solution-soaked cotton ball with sterile forceps.	
___	___	___	8. Cleanse the urinary meatus with one downward stroke, or use a circular motion from meatus to base of penis. Discard cotton ball. Repeat this step at least three to four times.	
___	___	___	9. Use forceps to pick up one dry cotton ball to dry the meatus.	
___	___	___	10. With sterile hand, pick up the catheter approximately 3 inches from the tip and lubricate catheter generously. (2% Lidocaine gel also can be applied.) Place distal catheter end into sterile basin.	
___	___	___	11. Gently insert catheter into urethra (approximately 8 inches) until urine begins to drain.	
___	___	___	12. Insert catheter an additional 1 inch (2.5 cm).	
___	___	___	13. If using an indwelling catheter, inflate the retention balloon with the prefilled syringe.	
___	___	___	14. Check for placement by gently pulling on catheter.	
___	___	___	15. Connect distal end of catheter to drainage bag if necessary.	
___	___	___	16. Tape catheter securely with 1-inch tape to the abdomen.	
___	___	___	17. In the uncircumcised male, gently replace the foreskin over the glans.	
___	___	___	18. Attach drainage bag to bed frame, coiling tubing to ensure that tubing does not fall into dependent loops.	
___	___	___	19. Wash hands.	

Excellent	Satisfactory	Needs Practice		Comments
			PROCEDURE 42-4 ## Inserting a Straight or Indwelling Urinary Catheter (*Continued*) **Goal:** To monitor urinary function, relieve bladder distension, provide continuous bladder drainage, obtain sterile urine specimen, or provide a means for irrigating the bladder.	
——	——	——	20. Record time of completion of procedure, size of catheter, amount and color of urine, and any adverse client responses.	
			Removing an Indwelling Catheter	
——	——	——	1. Wash hands.	
——	——	——	2. Don clean, disposable gloves.	
——	——	——	3. Clamp catheter (optional).	
——	——	——	4. Insert hub of syringe into balloon inflation tube of catheter, and draw out all liquid. Size of balloon is indicated on catheter; most commonly, sizes smaller than 10 mL are used. Larger balloons (30 mL) may be used after prostatic or urologic surgery.	
——	——	——	5. Ask client to breathe in and out deeply. Pinch gently and remove catheter as client exhales.	
——	——	——	6. Assist client to cleanse and dry genitals.	
——	——	——	7. Measure and document urine in drainage bag and time of catheter removal. Estimate when client should void (within 8 hours).	
——	——	——	8. Wash hands.	

Procedure Checklists to Accompany Craven and Hirnle's Fundamentals of Nursing: Human Health and Function, 5th edition

Name _____ Date _____

Unit _____ Position _____

Instructor/Evaluator: _____ Position _____

Excellent	Satisfactory	Needs Practice	PROCEDURE 43-1 **Assessing Stool for Occult Blood**	Comments
			Goal: To screen clients who have or are at risk for gastrointestinal bleeding.	
____	____	____	1. Identify client. Ask client to void before collecting stool specimen.	
____	____	____	2. Assist client onto bedpan, commode, or to bathroom. Provide privacy, and leave call bell within reach.	
____	____	____	3. When client has passed stool and is clean and comfortable, don disposable gloves, and obtain small amount of stool with tongue blade or wooden applicator.	
			Hemoccult Slide Test	
____	____	____	1. Open flap of slide, and apply a very thin smear of stool taken from center of the specimen onto first window.	
____	____	____	2. Using second applicator, obtain a second sample from a different area of stool. Smear thinly on second window of slide.	
____	____	____	3. Close slide cover. Wait 3–5 min., then open flap on reverse side, and apply two drops of Hemoccult developing solution onto each window and one drop to control window.	
____	____	____	4. Wait 30 to 60 seconds. Read test results.	
			Test With Hematest Tablets	
____	____	____	1. Apply small smear of stool onto guaiac filter paper.	
____	____	____	2. Place Hematest tablet on stool sample. Apply two to three drops of water onto Hematest tablet. Hold paper so water runs onto it.	
____	____	____	3. Read test results within 2 minutes by observing color of guaiac paper.	
____	____	____	4. Remove gloves, wash hands, and document findings.	

Procedure Checklists to Accompany Craven and Hirnle's Fundamentals
of Nursing: Human Health and Function, 5th edition

Name _____   Date _____

Unit _____   Position _____

Instructor/Evaluator: _____   Position _____

Excellent	Satisfactory	Needs Practice	PROCEDURE 43-2 **Administering an Enema**	Comments
			Goal: To relieve gas, constipation, or fecal impaction or to cleanse bowel in preparation for diagnostic tests.	
___	___	___	1. Assemble needed equipment in one place; then provide privacy by closing curtains or room door.	
___	___	___	2. Identify client. Position of left side (Sims' position) with right knee flexed.	
___	___	___	3. Put on disposable gloves. Place waterproof towel under client's buttocks.	
___	___	___	4. Cover client with bath blanket, exposing only the rectum.	
			Large-Volume Enema	
___	___	___	1. See Steps 1 to 4.	
___	___	___	2. Fill enema bag with 750 to 1000 mL lukewarm solution (105° to 110° F; for child, use 500 mL or less at 100° F). Check temperature of solution by pouring some over your inner wrist.	
___	___	___	3. Open clamp on tubing, and allow solution to flow through tubing to remove the air. Reclamp tubing.	
___	___	___	4. Lubricate 2 to 3 inches of tip of rectal tube with water-soluble lubricant.	
___	___	___	5. Separate the buttocks to visualize the anus. Observe for external hemorrhoids. Ask client to take a slow, deep breath. Gently insert the rectal tube, directing the tip toward the umbilicus (3–4 inches in the adult).	
___	___	___	6. Continue holding the tube in the rectum. With other hand, open the clamp and allow solution to slowly enter the client. Raise container 18 inches above the anus, allowing solution to flow slowly over 5 to 10 minutes. If client complains of cramping or pain, have client breathe deeply and lower bag until sensation stops.	
___	___	___	7. Reclamp tubing when desired amount of solution has infused.	
___	___	___	8. Remove tube gently and have client squeeze buttocks together firmly for several minutes.	

Excellent	Satisfactory	Needs Practice	

PROCEDURE 43-2
Administering an Enema (*Continued*)

Goal: To relieve gas, constipation, or fecal impaction or to cleanse bowel in preparation for diagnostic tests.

Comments

Excellent	Satisfactory	Needs Practice	Step
___	___	___	9. Have client retain solution as long as possible.
___	___	___	10. Assist client to bathroom, commode, or bedpan. Place call bell within reach. Provide privacy until all solution has been expelled.
___	___	___	11. Visually inspect character of the feces and solution. If client is to have enemas until clear, allow client to rest and then repeat as necessary.
___	___	___	12. Assist client into comfortable position. Assist with cleansing as needed. Provide materials for client to wash hands. Open windows or provide air freshener if needed. Clean and dispose of equipment as necessary. Remove gloves and wash hands.

Small-Volume Enema

Excellent	Satisfactory	Needs Practice	Step
___	___	___	1. See Steps 1 to 4 at beginning of procedure.
___	___	___	2. Remove protective cap from prelubricated catheter tip. You may add more lubricant if necessary.
___	___	___	3. Separate the buttocks to visualize the anus. Observe for hemorrhoids, and gently insert rectal tip into rectum, directing tip toward the umbilicus.
___	___	___	4. Squeeze bottle to empty contents into the rectum and colon (approximately 240 mL).
___	___	___	5. Maintain pressure on the enema container until you withdraw it from the rectum.
___	___	___	6. Continue same as with large-volume enema (see Steps 9 to 12).

Procedure Checklists to Accompany Craven and Hirnle's Fundamentals of Nursing: Human Health and Function, 5th edition

Name _____   Date _____

Unit _____   Position _____

Instructor/Evaluator: _____   Position _____

PROCEDURE 43-3
Inserting a Nasogastric Tube

Goal: To decompress the stomach to relieve pressure and prevent vomiting, to deliver enteral feedings, to provide a means to irrigate the stomach, or to obtain gastric specimen.

Excellent	Satisfactory	Needs Practice		Comments
____	____	____	1. Identify client and explain procedure.	
____	____	____	2. Provide privacy by closing curtains or room door. Raise bed to high Fowler's position, cover chest with towel, and place emesis basin nearby.	
____	____	____	3. Wash hands, and put on gloves. Determine length of tubing to be inserted by measuring nasogastric tube from tip of earlobe to tip of nose, then to tip of xiphoid process. Have client sit as straight as possible when measuring. If unable to sit up straight then take into consideration their slouched position when marking tube. Mark tubing with adhesive tape or note striped markings already on tube.	
____	____	____	4. Lubricate tip of tube with water-soluble lubricant.	
____	____	____	5. Gently insert tube into nostril. Advance toward posterior pharynx.	
____	____	____	6. Have client tilt head forward and encourage client to drink water slowly. Advance tube without using force as client swallows. Advance tube until desired insertion length is reached.	
____	____	____	7. Temporarily tape the tube to client's nose; then assess placement of tube:	
____	____	____	a. Aspirate gastric content with 20- to 50-mL syringe and test pH. If pH is less than 5, it can be assumed to be in the stomach.	
____	____	____	b. Though not supported by current evidence, some nurses carefully inject 10 to 20 mL air into nasogastric tube while auscultating over the epigastrium.	
____	____	____	c. If feeding tube is placed, x-ray confirmation of placement is required before any feeding is administered.	
____	____	____	8. If placement in stomach is not verified, untape tube, advance tube 5 cm, and repeat assessment in Step 7.	
____	____	____	9. Secure tube by taping to bridge of client's nose. Anchor tubing to client's gown.	

PROCEDURE 43-3
Inserting a Nasogastric Tube (*Continued*)

Excellent	Satisfactory	Needs Practice	**Goal:** To decompress the stomach to relieve pressure and prevent vomiting, to deliver enteral feedings, to provide a means to irrigate the stomach, or to obtain gastric specimen.	**Comments**
——	——	——	10. Clamp end of tubing or attach to suction, as ordered by health care provider.	
——	——	——	11. Wash hands, provide for client's comfort, and remove equipment.	
——	——	——	12. Establish and document a nursing plan for daily care of nasogastric tube:	
——	——	——	a. Inspect nostril for irritation.	
——	——	——	b. Cleanse nostril frequently.	
——	——	——	c. Change adhesive as required to prevent skin irritation or pressure sores on nostril from tube.	
——	——	——	d. Increase frequency of oral care because clients with nasogastric tubes often mouth breathe and may be NPO.	
——	——	——	13. Document procedure and observations.	

Procedure Checklists to Accompany Craven and Hirnle's Fundamentals of Nursing: Human Health and Function, 5th edition

Name _____ Date _____

Unit _____ Position _____

Instructor/Evaluator: _____ Position _____

Excellent	Satisfactory	Needs Practice	PROCEDURE 43-4 **Applying a Fecal Ostomy Pouch** **Goal:** To provide a means to contain drainage and odors from a fecal ostomy.	Comments
____	____	____	1. Identify client and provide privacy. Don disposable gloves. Client may perform procedure on self without gloves.	
____	____	____	2. Gently remove old appliance. If disposable, discard. If reusable, set aside for washing.	
____	____	____	3. Wash skin thoroughly around stoma with skin cleanser or soap and water.	
____	____	____	4. Rinse skin thoroughly and blot dry.	
____	____	____	5. Observe condition of peristomal skin, the stoma, and the sutures. Teach client to make these observations daily.	
____	____	____	6. Prepare clean pouch. Measure stoma and trace circle 1/8 inch larger than stoma on adhesive paper backing. Cut stoma pattern.	
____	____	____	7. Prepare skin barrier. Measure stoma and cut hole in barrier the same size as stoma. Be sure edges are rounded.	
____	____	____	8. If stoma is located in abdominal crease or skin is irregular, use paste barrier to fill the irregularity.	
____	____	____	9. Apply protective skin barrier. 　a. Peel paper backing off wafer and center stoma in hole. 　b. Place on abdomen, pressing lightly over all areas of the barrier to promote adhesion with skin surfaces.	
____	____	____	10. Attach drainable pouch to skin barrier. (Some equipment attaches by plastic flange that snaps in place; other models adhere through self-adherent tape that is exposed after protective paper backing is removed.) Tug gently or inspect for secure fit.	
____	____	____	11. Frame every edge of the faceplate with hypoallergenic tape.	
____	____	____	12. Fold over bottom edge of pouch and clamp.	
____	____	____	13. Dispose of old appliance. Clean and store any reusable supplies. Wash hands. Document noted observations.	

Procedure Checklists to Accompany Craven and Hirnle's Fundamentals of Nursing: Human Health and Function, 5th edition

Name _____ Date _____

Unit _____ Position _____

Instructor/Evaluator: _____ Position _____

Excellent	Satisfactory	Needs Practice		Comments
			PROCEDURE 45-1 **Pain Management: Epidural Analgesia** **Goal:** To administer medications via a patient-controlled epidural analgesia system.	
			Patient-Controlled Epidural Analgesia	
____	____	____	1. Check physician's order for current analgesia dose.	
____	____	____	2. Wash hands.	
____	____	____	3. Insert tubing into medication bag; prime tubing and filter. Place tubing in pump with proper rate set to deliver ordered dose. Set limit to amount of fluid in bag. Place epidural catheter label on tubing near pump.	
____	____	____	4. Cleanse connector of epidural catheter with Betadine. Wipe dry with sterile gauze.	
____	____	____	5. Remove cap from epidural catheter. Attach 3 mL syringe and aspirate. Moderate resistance will be felt. If more than 0.5 mL clear fluid or any blood is aspirated, STOP ASPIRATION. Remove syringe, recap catheter. Do not inject any fluid into catheter. Notify the anesthesia department immediately.	
____	____	____	6. If less than 0.5 mL fluid aspirated, remove syringe and connect tubing and filter to the client's epidural catheter. Confirm that all connections are secure. Confirm that epidural catheter label is in place on epidural catheter.	
____	____	____	7. Turn on pump and program per orders.	
			Patient-Controlled Epidural Analgesia (PCEA) with Continuous Infusion	
____	____	____	1. Repeat steps 1 to 6 above.	
____	____	____	2. a. Follow physician's order to load and increase infusion rate. Repeat per order.	
____	____	____	b. Notify physician if inadequate improvement in analgesia.	

Procedure Checklists to Accompany Craven and Hirnle's Fundamentals of Nursing: Human Health and Function, 5th edition

Name _____   Date _____

Unit _____   Position _____

Instructor/Evaluator: _____   Position _____

Excellent	Satisfactory	Needs Practice	PROCEDURE 45-2 ## Pain Management: Patient-Controlled Analgesia	Comments
			Goal: To allow clients to safely self-administer preset doses of prescribed analgesic intravenously.	
			Patient-Controlled Epidural Analgesia	
			Before beginning, check physician's orders.	

___ ___	___ ___	___ ___	1. Explain procedure to client:
			  a. Explain to visitiors/family that only the client is to use the "pain button."
			  b. Reinforce teaching throughout the course of therapy.
			  c. Document client and family teaching.	

___	___	___	2. Check IV site frequently for signs of infiltration or occlusion.	
___	___	___	3. If client is no longer capable of administering his or her medications, notify the physician.	
___	___	___	4. For problem-solving, refer to the trouble-shooting guide on the pump. The pain management nurse specialist and IV team also can help with problems related to the PCA infuser.	
___	___	___	5. A physician's order is required for discontinuation of the PCA infuser.	
___	___	___	6. Discard medication remaining in a syringe. Record action on computerized narcotic distribution cart. Another nurse must witness and enter into the record *wasted* drug.	
___	___	___	7. Record total medication dose (mg/mcg), milliliters (mL) infused, and milliliters (mL) left in Physical Assessment: Pain Assessment form EVERY SHIFT.	

*Procedure Checklists to Accompany Craven and Hirnle's Fundamentals
of Nursing: Human Health and Function,* 5th edition

Name _____ Date _____

Unit _____ Position _____

Instructor/Evaluator: _____ Position _____

Excellent	Satisfactory	Needs Practice	PROCEDURE 46-1 **Removing Contact Lenses**	Comments
			Goal: To remove contact lenses in the event the client is unable to do so.	
			Removing Hard Contact Lenses	
___	___	___	1. Wash hands with soap and warm water.	
___	___	___	2. Position client comfortably in sitting position if possible.	
___	___	___	3. Pull the client's upper and lower lid apart and pull tautly toward the lateral side.	
___	___	___	4. Ask client to blink, and the lens should pop out into your hand.	
___	___	___	5. Alternatively: Use lens suction cup, especially for clients who cannot consciously assist with removal.	
			Removing Soft Contact Lenses	
___	___	___	1. Wash hands with soap and warm water.	
___	___	___	2. Position client comfortably in a sitting position if possible.	
___	___	___	3. Ask client to look upward and inward. Pull down on the lower lid and place your index finger on the lower edge of the lens, moving it onto the white part of the eye.	
___	___	___	4. Gently grasp lens between thumb and index finger to release the suction of the lens. The lens will fold over and be easily removed. Gently roll the lens, using normal saline as needed, to separate the lens and return it to its normal form.	

Procedure Checklists to Accompany Craven and Hirnle's Fundamentals of Nursing: Human Health and Function, 5th edition

Name _____   Date _____

Unit _____   Position _____

Instructor/Evaluator: _____   Position _____

PROCEDURE 46-2
Assisting Adult with Inserting a Hearing Aid

Goal: To maintain hearing status by assisting with insertion of hearing aid.

Excellent	Satisfactory	Needs Practice		Comments
____	____	____	1. Check to be sure that the battery is functional. Hold hearing aid in hand and turn up the volume until you hear a "feedback" whistle.	
____	____	____	2. Inspect hearing aid to be sure that the tubing and ear mold are intact and not cracked or broken. The opening of the ear mold should be free of cerumen.	
____	____	____	3. With volume turned down, insert the ear mold into the ear canal, twisting slightly for a snug fit.	
____	____	____	4. Secure the battery behind the ear, if of that type. There are other styles of hearing aids that may fit in other ways.	
____	____	____	5. Turn the volume up slowly while speaking to the client in a normal voice tone. Ask client to let you know when the sound level is comfortable.	